Contents

PART 1: The Diet

PART 2: Meal Plan and Recipes

PART 3: How Does it Work?

PART 4: Where Are We Going?

PART 5: Ayurveda and Integrative Medicine for All Ages

PART I

The Diet

REST AND REPAIR DIET

CHAPTER 1

Beginnings

Samantha and I both experienced improvement in our digestion problems and gut health after 10 days on the Rest and Repair Diet. Weight loss has never been a concern for me but Samantha began the diet about 50 pounds above her ideal weight. She didn't think much about it, but after 9 months of being on the diet, she stepped on a scale and discovered that she had lost 50 pounds *without trying*. Since then she has used our Self Discovery program to fine-tune her weight. Most people think that they have to eat less and exercise more to lose weight and while this is true, it may not be enough because these changes don't take the condition of your gut into account.

The Rest and Repair diet is designed to detox your gut and allow it to repair itself, with weight loss as a side benefit. It takes advantage of the time-tested knowledge of Ayurveda, which emphasizes digestion as a vital aspect of health (see Chapter 6 for more on Ayurveda). *This diet makes use of your body's natural ability to heal itself and restore your microbiome.*

What exactly is the microbiome?

The microbiome consists of all the microorganisms (bacteria, fungi, viruses, etc.) that live *in* and *on* you. There are some 30 trillion microbes in your lower gut alone. The good news is that most of them are friendly.

Surprise! The state of your health depends upon the state of your gut bacteria. Most doctors and scientists understand that the gut bacteria have an enormous impact on both your mind and body, and that they may be key to the treatment of disorders and diseases—from diabetes to Alzheimer's, even obesity.

Hippocrates, who is considered to be the father of western medicine, said, "All disease begins in the gut." Conventional doctors used to consider this a strange concept, and even today cringe at the idea of another new diet fad.

Most alternative health experts, however, agree with Hippocrates. Some of them advocate a plant-based diet, with no meat or dairy. Others favor a Paleo diet, with no grains and lots of meat and fat. America is in the middle of the Diet War and there is no easy way to figure out which diet is best for your individual physiology.

What is the solution?

The same natural inner intelligence that runs the universe lies inside each human being. The problem is that in the name of "progress," you have gradually adopted bad habits, which disrupt your body and your mind and can eventually lead to chronic disease. Your physiology needs a chance to rest and repair itself and to re-enliven your own inner intelligence. This may sound simplistic, but it works.

Rest enables your body's repair systems to kick in and begin to heal and re-establish balance in your gut. Fatigue is the enemy.

How do you change a habit?

For one person, change is easy; for another, it can be hard. The Rest and Repair Diet is for everyone. It allows your body and mind to *clearly experience how each food affects you*. This feedback naturally reinforces your selection of the right food for your own nature or type, food that supports your microbiome rather than upsets it. The Rest and Repair Diet also promotes clearer awareness and sensitivity so that you can make other positive changes in your lifestyle.

THE REST AND REPAIR DIET

The Rest and Repair Diet is a simple step-by-step diet designed for both vegetarians and meat eaters to:

- Detoxify

- Heal the gut

- Improve digestion and health

- Lose weight

There are three phases to the Rest and Repair Diet:

- 1-Week Prep Detox Program

- 3-Week Rest and Repair Phase

- Self Discovery Lifestyle Program

How do you begin?

You begin with a week of detoxifying your body using simple herbal preparations and making a few easy changes in your lifestyle.

What's Next?

After your detox, you start the 3-Week Rest and Repair phase of the diet. We want you clearly understand that the Rest and Repair Diet is not a fast. Ideally, it should be a feast that improves your microbiome and digestion. Realistically, you should at least feel satisfied after each meal.

The Self Discovery Lifestyle Program

When you are finished with the Rest and Repair phase, you will then begin your Self Discovery Lifestyle Program. This is an important part of your road to health, and involves reintroducing specific foods eliminated in your 3-Week diet, as well as making appropriate long-term changes in your diet and lifestyle.

During this final phase, you will be keeping a *Food and Lifestyle Journal* so that it will be crystal clear how changes in food and lifestyle affect your body and mind.

What are the benefits of the Rest and Repair Diet?

The main benefit is to improve the state of your gut and make you generally healthier and more comfortable. Losing weight is an important side benefit. Obesity leads to many kinds of disorders, including diabetes and cardiovascular disease, the #1 killer in the modern world. You don't want to get too skinny, because that is not good for your health. You want to be strong, feel good, have energy, and maintain a healthy weight.

Okay. It's time to begin.

CHAPTER 2

The Rest And Repair Diet

WEEK 1

This ideal daily routine may seem like a big commitment, but positive changes in your lifestyle can actually help you stick to your diet!

DIET PREP DETOX

When You Wake Up

Drink a full glass of room temperature water and then use the bathroom for elimination.

Before Breakfast

- Meditate. We recommend the Transcendental Meditation® program. It only takes 20 minutes twice a day to bring positive changes to every aspect of your life—including your digestion (see tm.org).

- Exercise (even a simple morning walk)

- Yoga

Breakfast, Lunch, Dinner

- Wean yourself away from foods containing: gluten, dairy, and sugar (or artificial sweeteners).

- Your main meal of the day should be lunch. Sit comfortably in a stress-free environment, and stay sitting for a few minutes after the meal.

Throughout the Day

- Sip warm or hot water throughout the day and early evening.

- Three times a day, drink a traditional Digest and Detox Tea:

    - ½ teaspoon organic cumin

    - ½ teaspoon fennel

    - ½ teaspoon coriander seeds

    - 5 cups of hot water

- Boil this mixture for about 5 minutes, strain, and put in a thermos. (See Appendix 1 for this as a commercially available herbal product.)

- Before meals, especially lunch and dinner, prepare a pre-meal digestive aid, consisting of a mixture of fresh ginger juice, lemon juice, and a little salt. If it seems too strong to you, add a little water. To make the digestive aid:

  - Grate fresh raw organic ginger

  - Put the gratings in a piece of cheese cloth

  - Squeeze the juice into a small glass

  - Add lemon and salt to taste

- Avoid cold drinks (no ice) before, during, and after meals, because cold reduces your "digestive fire." You can sip small amounts of warm water with your meal and add a squeeze of lemon for taste.

Before Bed

To aid elimination, take the herbal preparation *triphala* with warm water, about 30-60 minutes before bed. (See Appendix 1 for triphala as a commercially available herbal product.)

Bedtime

Try to get to bed well before 10 pm to have a good night's sleep. (It will help if you start getting ready a half an hour before.)

WEEKS 2, 3, and 4

THE REST AND REPAIR DIET

1. Continue with Week 1 Diet Prep Detox Program.

2. This is the time to eliminate all gluten-containing foods. We have found a few good tasting commercial gluten-free breads and pastas, as well as gluten-free mixes for crepes and waffles, which we predict will soon be welcome in your dietary routine. (See Chapter 4 for Recipes)

3. Eliminate all dairy products containing lactose. Since lassi, yogurt, butter, ghee, and some cheeses contain only small amounts of lactose, moderate amounts may be included in your diet. (See Recipes)

4. Eliminate sugar and artificial sweeteners. You can use stevia or small amounts of maple syrup, coconut sugar, jaggery, or honey. According to traditional health systems, high heating changes honey's chemical makeup and can cause problems, so please don't cook the honey. Jaggery is a traditional sweetener used in Asia, which is usually processed from concentrated sugarcane juice, and contains additional vitamins and minerals. (If you are diabetic, make sure to check with your doctor since most of these sweeteners can raise blood sugar levels).

5. See the Meal Plan (next chapter) for a sample of Breakfast, Lunch, and Dinner menus. For lunch and dinner, it's best for both veggie and meat eaters to include a special food called kitchari at least once a day. (See Recipes) Kitchari is a mixture of rice and dhal and is used in Ayurveda to heal the gut and improve digestion. (Ayurveda—see Chapter 6)

6. For meat eaters and for flexible vegetarians, bone broth is a traditional time-tested remedy to help heal your gut lining. Drink 1 cup of Chicken Bone Broth 3 times daily. (See Recipes) Meat eaters should eliminate red meat during the few weeks of this diet but chicken or fish can be included.

7. Cravings may arise (especially for sugar).

8. First, don't bring any food into your house that isn't good for you (and don't let anyone else do it either). The less temptation, the better.

9. Second, if you find yourself in the merciless claws of a craving, it is time for Damage Control. Ask yourself, "What can I eat right now that will give me satisfaction and cause the least damage to my health?" (See Meal Plan for snacks)

10. Third and finally, if you still can't subdue your cravings, try ½ teaspoon each of the medicinal herbs Ashwagandha and Brahmi. (See Appendix 1 for these as commercially available herbal products.)

11. These particular herbs are adaptogens, which are calming to your mind and emotions, and help you deal with stress

and change. Take the Ashwagandha and Brahmi together with warm water in the morning, late afternoon, and again in the evening. (If you suffer from hyperthyroidism check with your medical adviser to be sure that this is suitable for your situation.)

12. If you feel that you are not getting enough protein, add a protein shake to your diet. (See Recipes)

13. Our Meal Plan is designed to give you variety as well as nourishment and we have included delicious options. Try to be creative so that your food boredom is minimal.

14. For best results, emotionally and physically, identify a buddy who can encourage and commiserate with you. Check with your buddy every day and compare experiences. If you are doing the diet alone, be kind and patient with yourself.

SELF DISCOVERY LIFESTYLE PROGRAM

1. The Self Discovery Lifestyle Program is the final and perhaps most important part of the Rest and Repair Diet because it involves reintroducing foods you have eliminated in the past 3 weeks, noting their effect in a food journal, and using that information to make positive changes in your diet and lifestyle.

2. Ease yourself back into your new "normal" diet very gradually. Introduce gluten products, dairy, and sugar one at a

time, so that you can become aware of your body and mind's response to each food. Note that it can take a while for your physiology to be able to handle different foods. If you don't feel so good when you reintroduce something, try again in about 10 days. If you are still uncomfortable, then this food is probably not right for your individual physiology.

3. Take a daily probiotic either in the form of a capsule or a drink. You can include natural probiotics such as yogurt, lassi, etc. Fresh homemade yogurt is (of course) preferable to store bought commercial yogurts, which are necessarily old and often contain large quantities of sugar.

4. Take our Free Online Gut/Brain Quiz to learn the best foods for your own Gut/Brain Nature. (Go to Quiz at docgut.com.) The quiz also offers personalized lifestyle recommendations to help keep you in balance. (Lists of foods that are best for your Gut/Brain Nature are in the Chapter 21.)

5. Continue with your Ayurvedic daily routine which includes: drinking a full glass of room temperature water when you wake up and then elimination; meditating, exercising, and yoga before breakfast; having your main meal of the day at lunch. To aid elimination, take the herbal preparation triphala with warm water, about 30-60 minutes before bed; try to get to bed well before 10 pm and have a good night's sleep.

6. Awareness or attention is key to making positive changes in your life. It's not easy to give up ingrained habits and

addictions, and it helps to make changes in small steps, with your full attention.

7.   Positivity and support from friends and family will make your journey to gut health easier and happier. Try to communicate with them how important the process is to you, and celebrate milestones together.

8.   Be adaptable. Whenever you are eating out, for instance, be careful (also tactful and polite) and as best you can, avoid eating foods that are not on your diet. When you travel, it can be hard to find the right kinds of food, so be proactive and bring along plenty of nutritious snacks and teas. This might not be convenient, but you will feel a lot better when you reach your destination.

9.   *Your Healthy Gut* is an online course, offered by Maharishi University of Management, which carefully guides you through the Rest and Repair Diet, and connects you on Facebook with other people who are also on the diet.

10.   Your Food and Lifestyle Journal: Buy a handy size journal and keep it nearby to make notes on how you are feeling physically and mentally as you gradually re-introduce different foods each week or two. This will help you identify which culprits upset your system.

Journal Tips

- Be specific. For instance, when Samantha reintroduced oats, she was surprised to have unpleasant symptoms, which she described in her journal. (Gluten-free oats are available.)

- Written or digital? Some of us like to write in a little book, others prefer technology.

- Keep your journal handy, either beside your bed, on the table, or in your pocket.

- Be true to your own experience and honest about how you are feeling. Accept your reality—no one is judging.

- If an overwhelming craving knocks you off the diet, just write the facts down in a few words and start again.

- Compare notes with your buddy.

General Questions and Answers

Should I consult my doctor?

Before beginning this or any other diet, please consult your doctor, especially if you have a serious health condition. This diet should not even be considered by anyone who is weak or thin, or for young children. We don't want any part of the diet to interfere with your normal medical treatment.

Should I continue with my vitamin and mineral supplements, herbal supplements, or probiotics?

Yes. Especially if recommended by your doctor.

How long do I have to stay on the main diet phase?

Aim for 3 weeks. But if you can't continue after 2 weeks, then do as much as is comfortable. Even a week or 10 days will bring you some benefit.

I am a mom and too busy to do everything in the daily routine. What should I focus on?

Focus on the Rest and Repair Diet since it will improve your digestion and gut health.

What if I go off the diet?

Don't worry. Simply pick it up again and continue. You can do what you can do.

What if I lose too much weight?

If you are not overweight to start with, and find that you are losing more than two pounds a week, be sure to add lots of beneficial oils like ghee and olive and coconut oil, along with nutritious nuts, seeds, and avocados, to each meal.

Can I have raw vegetable juices during the Rest and Repair Diet?

No. This is one time to avoid all raw vegetables, including salads. Raw vegetables are much harder to digest and it is important to give your gut at least this period to repair itself.

Should I stop caffeine and alcohol?

It is best to eliminate caffeine (or at least greatly reduce), but do it slowly if you know you are addicted. You may have a small amount of alcohol (1/2 cup of red wine a day but no beer because it contains gluten.)

I am a vegetarian. Is it okay for me to try the bone broth?

If you are a strict vegetarian you would avoid it, but if you are a flexible vegetarian then it is okay.

I am a vegetarian but I am allergic to rice. What should I do?

Avoid it. Either substitute another non-gluten grain, or have the dhal by itself.

I am a vegetarian but I can't handle any kind of beans. What should I do?

Mung dhal is a legume, not a bean, and is very easy to digest. If you can't handle mung dhal, have rice soup cooked with a few vegetables.

How do I get enough protein?

Kitchari includes both mung dhal and rice. Mung dhal is a quality protein (1 cup cooked mung provides 14 grams of protein). Taken with rice, it forms a complete protein. Mung dhal also contains valuable nutrients like magnesium, B vitamins, manganese, and zinc.

Your body can only absorb and process about 20 grams of protein at one meal, so it's best to spread your protein intake over several meals. If you are worried about not getting enough protein, include a daily protein shake or eggs in your diet (see Meal Plans and Recipes). Two organic eggs provides 15 grams of high quality protein.

Which is better, green whole dhal or split yellow?

They are both fine, and both are called "mung dhal." One is yellow split mung, with the skin taken off. The other is green mung that still has the skin and, therefore, requires soaking before cooking.

What are the best probiotics?

Not all probiotics are equally effective, so it's important to evaluate them and then experiment to see which works best for you. See the Probiotic Rating Chart at docgut.com. (https://docgut.com/docguts-probiotic-rating/).

What kinds of food are allowed on the Rest and Repair Diet?

- Most fresh or frozen vegetables are good, with the exception of foods that are hard to digest or which produce gas. (See Chapter 21.)

- Most fresh or frozen fruits are acceptable.

- Most legumes are acceptable. But since you are already having mung dhal once a day, you might not want to add more.

- Most nuts are acceptable, but avoid canned mixes since they often contain food additives.

- Most spices are acceptable, but you don't want to use something that bothers your stomach.

- Some dairy products are acceptable, such as yogurt, butter, ghee, and lassi. Panir and goat cheese should be eaten in moderation.

- Eggs can be included for both flexible vegetarians and meat eaters.

- Meat eaters can have chicken and fish, but should avoid red meat, pork, and processed meats.

Do we have to use only organic products?

During this detox diet especially, you don't want to take in unnecessary toxins. This is the reason we recommend that all ingredients are organic and non-GMO. Use filtered or bottled drinking water whenever possible. And avoid canned foods since they usually contain added sugars, processing aids, and preservative chemicals.

When should I do the 3-Week Rest and Repair Diet again?

We suggest doing this diet once a year, especially at the beginning of spring.

PART 2

Meal Plan and Recipes

REST AND REPAIR DIET

CHAPTER 3

Meal Plan

We offer you two different meal plans for the 3 weeks of the Rest and Repair Diet. The first is the Basic Plan for those who prefer a purely Ayurvedic diet, designed to detox your body and reboot digestive fire. The second is the Variety Plan for if you want a wider ranger of choices that include both Ayurveda and other recipes.

Basic Plan for all 3 Weeks of the Rest and Repair Diet

The foundation of the Rest and Repair Diet is a traditional Ayurvedic Spring Detox Diet, which we call the Basic Plan. It consists of stewed apples for breakfast, with kitchari and cooked vegetables for lunch and dinner. In Chapter 4, you will find recipes and ways of preparing these basic meals, that will help reduce your shopping and cooking time.

	MONDAY	TUESDAY	WEDNESDAY
BREAKFAST	Stewed Apples	Stewed Apples	Stewed Apples
LUNCH	Kitchari + Cooked Veggies	Kitchari + Cooked Veggies	Kitchari + Cooked Veggies
SNACK	See Options Below	See Options Below	See Options Below
DINNER	Kitchari and/or Soup	Kitchari and/or Soup	Kitchari and/or Soup
OPTIONS	Chicken Bone Broth 3 times a day	Chicken Bone Broth 3 times a day	Chicken Bone Broth 3 times a day

Thursday	*Friday*	*Saturday*	*Sunday*
Stewed Apples	Stewed Apples	Stewed Apples	Stewed Apples
Kitchari + Cooked Veggies	Kitchari + Cooked Veggies	Kitchari + Cooked Veggies	Kitchari + Cooked Veggies
See Options Below	See Options Below	See Options Below	See Options Below
Kitchari and/or Soup	Kitchari and/or Soup	Kitchari and/or Soup	Kitchari and/or Soup
Chicken Bone Broth 3 times a day	Chicken Bone Broth 3 times a day	Chicken Bone Broth 3 times a day	Chicken Bone Broth 3 times a day

Variety Plan for the Rest and Repair Diet

We realize that the Basic Plan might be boring, so we have added the Variety Plan, which consists of two different categories: Simple Meals for people who don't have the time or inclination to cook, and Specialty Meals for those who enjoy cooking and have time to prepare a more elaborate meal.

Meat eaters can add chicken and fish throughout the three weeks of the diet. (We don't include recipes for chicken or fish.) Our only guideline is to make sure the recipes you use are gluten-free (GF), dairy-free, and with only the sweeteners we recommend.

WEEK ONE

	MONDAY	TUESDAY	WEDNESDAY
BREAKFAST	Sautéed Apples with Almond 35 Tortilla	Toast with Almond Butter	Chia Pudding Parfait with Fruit, Nuts, and Seeds
LUNCH	Kitchari + Cooked Veggies	Kitchari + Twice Baked Sweet Potatoes with Coconut Oil and Cinnamon	Kitchari + Vietnamese Spring Roll with Dipping Sauce
SNACK	Babaganoush with GF Crackers or Veggies	Spring Dip with GF Crackers	GF Zucchini Cake with Ghee and Honey
DINNER	Indian Dahl Soup	Rice or Pasta and Cooked Veggies	Vegan Creamy Asparagus and Pea Soup

You can tailor your own 3-week meal plan to your preference and lifestyle. In Chapter 4, we include a variety of recipes and options for breakfast, snacks, soups, and other meals. On the Variety Plan, you only need to have kitchari once a day.

*You can add toppers to the soup, such as crispy shallots, capers, yogurt, or toasted nuts or seeds. Feel free to mix and match or stick to the traditional kitchari meal plan. Enjoy!

THURSDAY	FRIDAY	SATURDAY	SUNDAY
Egg Scramble with Avocado	Golden Milk	Granola	Gluten Free Waffles
Kitchari + GF Enchiladas	Kitchari + Macro Lunch Bowl	Kitchari + Avocado Sushi	Kitchari + Vegan Green Bean Casserole
Rice Cakes and Avocado	Vegan Avocado Crema with Baked Zucchini Chips	Spring Dip with GF Crackers	Maple Almond Cookies
Tortilla Soup	Rice or Pasta and Cooked Veggies	Tuscan White Bean and Kale Soup with Rosemary and Parsley	Minestrone Soup

WEEK TWO

	MONDAY	TUESDAY	WEDNESDAY
BREAKFAST	Sautéed Apples with Roasted Potatoes	Protein Shake	Crispy Haystacks
LUNCH	Kitchari + Roasted Fennel With Preserved Lemons and GF Breadcrumbs	Kitchari + Polenta Cake with Sautéed Veggies and Tomato Confit	Kitchari + Asian Pasta and Veggies Bowl
SNACK	Guacamole with Veggies and/or GF Tortilla Chips	Chocolate Avocado Mousse	GF Cornbread
DINNER	Indian Dhal Soup	Rice or Pasta and Cooked Veggies	Vegan Creamy Asparagus and Pea soup

WEEK THREE

	MONDAY	TUESDAY	WEDNESDAY
BREAKFAST	Stewed Apples	Egg Scramble with Avocado	Granola
LUNCH	Kitchari + Vegan Green Bean Casserole	Kitchari + Roasted Fennel With Preserved Lemons And GF Breadcrumbs	Kitchari + Faux Ahi Tuna and Avocado Salsa
SNACK	4 Ingredient Almond Maple Cookies with Golden Milk	Roasted Beet and White Bean Hummus with GF Crackers or Veggies	Crispy Chickpeas
DINNER	Indian Dhal Soup	Rice or Pasta and Cooked Veggies	Vegan Creamy Asparagus and Pea soup

THURSDAY	FRIDAY	SATURDAY	SUNDAY
Toast with Almond Butter	Stewed Apples	Egg Scramble with Avocado	GF Crepes
Kitchari + Avocado Sushi	Kitchari + Vegan/ GF Green Bean Casserole	Kitchari + Zucchini Gratin	Kitchari + GF Enchiladas
Guacamole with Veggies and/or GF Tortilla Chips	GF Cornbread	Chocolate Avocado Mousse	Guacamole with Veggies and/or GF Tortilla Chips
Tortilla soup	Rice or Pasta and Cooked Veggies	Tuscan White Bean & Kale Soup with Rosemary and Parsley	Minestrone Soup

THURSDAY	FRIDAY	SATURDAY	SUNDAY
Fresh Fruit	Golden Milk	Chia Pudding Parfait with Fruit, Nuts, and Seeds	GF French Toast
Kitchari + Macro Lunch	Kitchari + Zucchini Gratin	Kitchari + Crispy Haystacks	Kitchari + GF Mediterranean Pasta and Veggies
Roasted Beet and White Bean Hummus with GF Crackers or Veggies	4 Ingredient Almond Maple Cookies with Golden Milk	Crispy chickpeas	Roasted Beet and White Bean Hummus with GF Crackers or Veggies
Tortilla soup	Rice or Pasta and Cooked Veggies	Tuscan White Bean & Kale Soup with Rosemary and Parsley	Minestrone Soup

CHAPTER 4

Recipes

THE BASIC PLAN

Breakfast

STEWED APPLES/PEARS WITH CINNAMON AND GINGER
(Alexis Farley and Andrew Stenberg)

Time:

20 minutes (prep 10 minutes, cooking 10 minutes)

Serves:

1-2

Ingredients:

½ -3 cups water

½ cinnamon stick or 1 teaspoon ground cinnamon

1 inch fresh grated ginger, or ¾ teaspoon powdered ginger

2 apples, peeled, cored, and halved (pears optional)

2 tablespoons chopped toasted walnuts or almonds

8 cloves

A little sweetener (e.g. maple syrup or jaggery)

Directions:

1. Peel and core apples and cut into quarters. Push one clove into each quarter (take the cloves out before you eat). You can pears with the apples, stewed with cloves.

2. Boil the water with all the ingredients. Reduce the heat to Low and cover until the apples are soft (5 minutes). During cooking, add a small amount of cardamom and cinnamon powder. Also add freshly grated ginger or ginger powder.

3. Remove and sprinkle with walnuts or blanched almonds.

Note:

You can also add Flame or Thompson raisins, and/or dried apricots, and/or Medjool dates–but not too many!

You can puree this mixture, but remove the cloves first, as their taste can be a bit strong. Also, be VERY CAREFUL if you puree a hot mixture in a machine! It is better to carefully use a blending wand.

Lunch and Dinner

KITCHARI 1
(Alexis)

Time:

60 minutes (prep 20 minutes, cooking 40 minutes)

*soak beans overnight

Serves:

4

Ingredients:

½ cup split yellow mung beans (washed and presoaked)

½ cup white basmati rice (washed)

2 tablespoons coconut oil or ghee

4 cups homemade vegetable stock or water

2 tablespoons coconut cream

1½ teaspoons cumin seeds

1½ teaspoons fennel seeds

1½ teaspoons coriander powder

1 tablespoon ginger root (peeled and minced)

½ teaspoon turmeric powder

½ teaspoon fenugreek seeds

¼ teaspoon black mustard seeds

⅛ teaspoon asafoetida

2 cups of any mixed vegetables with maximum of 3 vegetables
of digestion (optional)

1 lime (juiced)

⅓ cup yogurt

sea salt to taste

Directions:

1. The night before (24 hours earlier), soak mung beans in water

2. When you're ready to cook, drain the mung beans and rinse
    under running water. Place rice in a sieve and rinse till the
    water runs clear.

3. Prepare vegetables by peeling and chopping them up, then
    set aside. This is the time to peel and dice the ginger.

4. In a large pot heat coconut oil or ghee over Medium heat.

5. Add cumin, fennel, fenugreek and black mustard seeds and
    cook for a few minutes until the mustard seeds have popped.
    Add the rest of the spices and stir to combine.

6. Add 1 cup of vegetable stock or water, mung beans, coconut
    cream, rice and vegetables, then add the remaining 3 cups of
    stock or water.

7. Cover and bring to a boil, then reduce to a low heat. Simmer
    for about 40 minutes. Check the pot periodically because the
    rice swells and may stick to the bottom.

8. Add more water for a soupier consistency. Simmer longer to get a thicker stew.

9. Serve with a squeeze of fresh lime juice, spoonful of yogurt, and sea salt to taste.

KITCHARI 2
(Andrew)

Time:

30 minutes (less time with pressure cooker)

*soak beans overnight

Serves:

2 - 3

Ingredients:

½ cup split yellow mung beans (washed and presoaked)

½ cup white basmati rice (washed)

2½ to 3 cups of water

1 teaspoon cumin seeds

¼ teaspoon fenugreek seeds

¼ teaspoon fennel seeds

¼ teaspoon ajwan seeds

¼ teaspoon mustard seeds

½ teaspoon ginger

1 teaspoon turmeric

1 teaspoon coriander

½ teaspoon salt

lemon juice

vegetables and nuts (optional)

Directions:

1. Wash rice and mung dhal, soak overnight.

2. Drain water.

3. Put the whole spices in one small bowl, and the powdered spices in another, so that you can add them to the ghee at different times.

4. Heat 1 tablespoon of ghee in a pan. When the temperature is hot enough, the seeds should pop when you drop them into the ghee. Allow them to simmer for a little while before adding in the powdered spices. Stir and let the mixture cook for a minute or two, or until the aroma becomes noticeable. Don't let them burn!

5. Add the rice and mung dhal and sauté for another couple of minutes. Then add water and bring to a boil.

6. Once the kitchari is boiling, reduce the heat to Medium-Low. Cover and cook until it is tender (20 - 30 minutes).

7. If needed, add more water. Tastes vary and some people like it thinner, some a little thicker.

8. Before serving, you can add a little lemon juice and extra salt and pepper to taste.

Note 1:

If you are adding vegetables into the kitchari, add the longer cooking vegetables, such as carrots and beets, halfway through cooking. Add vegetables that cook faster, such as leafy greens, about 5 minutes before the end. Add more water as needed.

Garnish with fresh cilantro and add salt to taste (optional).

Nuts and/or seeds (preferably soaked and chopped) can be added at the end of the cooking.

Nuts: almonds, walnuts, cashews, pine nuts, macadamia nuts

Seeds: pumpkin seeds, sunflower seeds, chia seeds, ground flaxseed.

Note 2:

You can use a pressure cooker, which, of course, is much faster. Combine ingredients and cook for 3-4 minutes after the pressure has built up.

An easy way to make kitchari in the morning is to boil the same ingredients (except for lemon) for a few minutes and then place in a large thermos. It will then continue cooking in the thermos and can be eaten at lunch and should still be hot.

KITCHARI 3
(Dolores Johnson)

Time:

30 minutes

*soak beans and rice overnight

Serves:

2 - 3

Ingredients:

¼ cup rice

½ cup split yellow mung beans

2½ to 3 cups of water

½ teaspoon fennel seed

½ teaspoons whole cumin seeds

½ teaspoons cumin powder

½ teaspoon coriander

cinnamon or cardamom – a pinch

ghee for cooking spices

salt to taste

dash of lemon juice

1 cup chopped assorted vegetables

Directions:

1. Rinse dhal and check for stones, soak overnight.

2. Rinse rice, soak overnight.

3. When ready to cook drain water off dhal and rice.

4. Add rice and dhal to 2½ to 3 cups of water.

5. Add fennel seeds and bring to a boil.

6. Cover and lower the temperature to medium low.

7. While the dhal/rice is cooking heat the ghee.

8. Toast the whole cumin until it is toasted-be carefully not to burn.

9. Add the cumin powder and then add to the dhal/ rice mixture.

10. Add pinch of cinnamon or cardamom, salt to dhal/rice.

11. Add vegetables (if using).

12. Depending on how thick you like the kitchari, you may want to add more water.

13. Cover and cook until tender (25-30 minutes.)

14. Before serving add lemon juice and chopped fresh cilantro.

Good for All Plans for Meat Eaters and Optional for Vegetarians:

CHICKEN BONE BROTH
(adapted from Dr. Maggie)

Time:

12 to 48 hours

Serves:

1-2

* soak chicken bones in apple cider vinegar and cold water one hour before cooking

Ingredients:

3-6 pounds chicken bones

¼ cup apple cider vinegar

8-10 quarts of water (depending on the size of the crock pot)

1 tablespoon Himalayan pink sea salt

Directions:

1. It is easiest to use a slow cooker to properly prepare the broth. The bones are placed in cold water with apple cider vinegar for one hour ahead of time.

2. Add water and salt and cook on Low in a crock pot for 12-48 hours (longer the better). Strain out the solid ingredients.

3. Once the broth has cooled to room temperature, store the broth in a glass container (bowl) in the refrigerator.

4. When it is cold it will look like jello. If it does not, then the next time you will need to add more bones or less water. Do not discard your bones. You may use the same bones up to three times for cooking or drinking.

Note:

The difference between chicken broth and chicken stock is that the stock is a mixture of meat and water. If you add vegetables it becomes a stew. As an alternative, good-quality chicken bone broth can be purchased – just make sure that it is organic.

If you can, take a cup 3 times a day with meals.

<u>VARIETY PLAN: FIRST, SIMPLE MEALS</u>

Breakfast

TOAST AND ALMOND OR OTHER NUT BUTTER
(Samantha & Keith)

Time:

  5 minutes

Serves:

  1-2

Ingredients:

  gluten-free bread

  roasted nut butter (organic if possible)

Directions:

1. Toast the bread.

2. Optional: add ghee.

3. Spread with your choice of nut butter (Ayurveda does not recommend peanuts).

FRIED APPLES WITH POTATOES
"HEAVEN AND EARTH"
(Samantha & Keith)

Time:

10 minutes (boil potatoes the night before and refrigerate)

Serves:

1-2

Ingredients:

2-3 apples peeled

2-3 potatoes boiled and then fried

2 tablespoons ghee

salt and pepper

avocado and lemon (optional)

Directions:

1. Cut up potatoes and fry until brown.

2. Peel and slice apples.

3. Fry potatoes a little longer than apples in one pan with ghee until slightly brown at the edges.

4. Fry apples in another pan with ghee until edges are golden brown on each side.

5. While frying, often turn over the potatoes and apples

6. Once cooked, mix together.

7. Add salt and pepper to taste.

8. Optional: Add avocado and lemon.

Note:

As an alternative to the potatoes we often enjoy roasted and salted pecans and walnuts.

FRIED APPLES WITH READY-MADE GLUTEN-FREE ALMOND TORTILLA
(Samantha & Keith)

Time:

10 minutes

Serves:

2

Ingredients:

2-3 apples peeled
2 gluten-free almond tortillas

Directions:

1. Peel and slice up apples

2. Fry in pan with ghee until slightly brown on each side

3. Fry gluten-free tortilla

4. Optional: Serve with jam (organic black current jam is fabulous with this dish)

Note:

We like the Siete brand of almond tortilla, although it is expensive. And we enjoy Crofter's black current jam, which is reasonably priced.

COOKED OATMEAL
(Andrew)

Time:

10 minutes

Serves:

1-2

Ingredients:

gluten-free oatmeal

raisins, cardamom, cinnamon and ginger

Directions:

1. Follow directions on gluten-free oatmeal package.

2. Add raisins, cardamom, cinnamon, and ginger to taste.

Note:

You can mix whey, or brown rice or hemp seed protein powder into the oatmeal, etc. if you like – it is a tasty way to get about 20 grams of protein in an easily-digestible form.

EGGS (ANY STYLE)

As we mentioned, for egg-eaters, a couple of organic eggs will be fine for breakfast while you are on this diet.

REHEATED KITCHARI

You can heat leftover kitchari from the night before for breakfast, as long as it has been refrigerated overnight. It's not ideal to eat leftovers, but this is a good high-protein, digestible breakfast for anyone in a hurry (you can add nuts or raisins).

PROTEIN SHAKE

Simply blend together 8 ounces water (or unsweetened organic almond, hazelnut, or rice milk) and the desired amount of protein powder of your choice, along with a pinch of cardamom and cinnamon. You can also add fruit and/or seeds, along with honey or stevia.

Lunch or Dinner

RICE AND VEGGIES
(Samantha & Keith)

Time:

35 minutes (prep 10 minutes, cooking 15 minutes, let stand 10 minutes)

Serves:

1-2

Ingredients:

½ cup basmati rice

1 cup water

Veggies and spices of your choice, depending on your Gut/Brain Nature (see Chapter 22).

Directions:

1. Clean rice.

2. Boil water, add rice, and let simmer for 15 minutes. If you are using a rice cooker, follow instructions.

3. If you are using the stove top method, bring to a boil, reduce the heat and simmer (covered) for 15 minutes. Remove from heat and let stand (covered) for another 10 minutes before fluffing with a fork.

4. Steam, roast, or sauté vegetables.

5. Add spices when cooking.

6. Add salt and pepper to taste.

QUICK MEDITERRANEAN PASTA
(Samantha & Keith)

Time:

10 minutes

Serves:

2

Ingredients:

4-8 ounces gluten-free pasta of your choice (depending on serving size)

1 tablespoon olive oil or ghee

3 orange peppers

6 mushrooms of your choice

6 ounces tomato sauce in glass jar

6 ounces unsweetened coconut cream (or to taste)

Directions:

1. Wash and slice 1 or 2 orange peppers into two-inch pieces.

2. Clean mushrooms with a rough cloth or brush or paper towels and slice.

3. Sauté orange peppers, and only add the mushrooms about 5 minutes before the end (they cook more quickly).

4. Bring a pot of water to a boil and follow product directions to cook gluten-free pasta.

5. Add tomato sauce or non-dairy gluten-free sauce of your choice.

Note:

We add unsweetened coconut cream to tomato sauce to make a less acidic and richer pink sauce.

QUICK ASIAN PASTA
(Samantha & Keith)

Time:

10 minutes

Serves:

1-2

Ingredients:

4-8 ounces of gluten-free pasta of your choice (depending on serves size)

2 yellow squash or zucchini

6 mushrooms of your choice

gluten-free tamari (optional)

toasted sesame oil (optional)

Directions:

1. Follow product directions to cook gluten-free pasta.

2. In a separate pan, sauté yellow squash or zucchini, and add the mushrooms halfway through.

3. Add gluten-free tamari and/or toasted sesame oil to taste.

AVOCADO SANDWICH
(Samantha & Keith)

Time:

10 minutes

Serves:

1-2

Ingredients:

1 avocado

ghee or olive oil to taste

lemon to taste

salt and pepper to taste

Directions

1. Toast gluten-free bread.

2. Spread ghee or olive oil on toast.

3. Add sliced or mashed avocado.

4. Season with lemon, salt and pepper.

Soups

CREAMY ASPARAGUS AND PEA SOUP
(Adapted from Minimalist Baker recipe)

Time:

30 minutes total (5 minutes prep, 25 minutes cooking)

Serves:

2-3

Ingredients:

2 tablespoons olive or avocado oil

12 ounces asparagus (1 large bundle yields 12 ounces)

10 ounces fresh or frozen peas (2 cups yield 10 ounces)

4 cloves garlic (optional)

1 medium shallot (thinly sliced)

1½ cups plain almond milk (must be unsweetened)

1½ cups vegetable broth

¼ teaspoon cardamom or to taste

¼ teaspoon coriander or to taste

cinnamon – a pinch or to taste

salt and pepper to taste

½ medium size lemon (optional)

Directions:

1. Preheat oven to 400 degrees F and spread asparagus on a bare baking sheet. Drizzle with oil of choice and season lightly with salt and pepper. Toss to coat.

2. Roast for 15 minutes, then set aside.

3. Heat a large saucepan or medium pot. Once hot, add 2 tablespoons oil, shallot, and garlic. Season lightly with salt and pepper, and stir to coat. Cook for 2-3 minutes or until fragrant and translucent. Reduce heat if garlic begins to brown.

4. Add vegetable broth and almond milk. Season with salt and pepper once more.

5. Transfer soup to blender along with asparagus (reserve some asparagus for garnish if desired). Blend soup until creamy and smooth. Transfer back to pot and bring to Medium heat and simmer.

6. Taste and adjust seasonings as needed. Remove from heat and squeeze the lemon over the soup.

1-POT VEGAN GLUTEN-FREE MINESTRONE
(Adapted from Minimalist Baker)

Time:

30 minutes (prep 5 minutes, cook 25 minutes)

Serves:

6

Ingredients:

2 tablespoons water (you can substitute olive oil)

½ medium white or yellow onion (diced)

3 cloves garlic (minced)

2 large carrots (peeled and sliced into thin rounds)

1½ cups green beans (trimmed and roughly chopped)

¼ teaspoon each sea salt and black pepper (plus more to taste)

1 small zucchini (sliced into 1/4-inch rounds)

5 or 6 whole tomatoes, peeled and diced

6 cups vegetable broth

2 teaspoons dried basil

2 teaspoons dried oregano

1 teaspoon coconut sugar or other sweetener (optional to taste)

2 cups gluten-free pasta noodles

1 cup kale, spinach, or other greens (roughly chopped)

Directions:

1. Heat a large pot or Dutch oven over Medium heat. Once hot, add water, onions, and garlic. Cook for 3 minutes, stirring occasionally.

2. Add carrots and green beans and season with salt and pepper. Cook for 3-4 minutes, stirring occasionally, until vegetables have softened slightly and have some color.

3. Add zucchini, tomatoes, vegetable broth, basil, and oregano. Stir to coat.

4. Increase heat to Medium-High and bring soup to a strong simmer. Then reduce heat slightly to Medium-Low until the soup is simmering but not boiling.

5. Add pasta and stir. Cook for 10 minutes, stirring occasionally. Reduce heat if needed to keep the soup at a simmer.

6. Reduce heat to Low and simmer for 4-5 minutes, stirring occasionally. Taste soup and adjust seasonings as needed, adding coconut sugar to balance the flavors (optional).

7. Add kale or spinach (or other greens) and stir. Cook for another 3-4 minutes to wilt the kale and allow the flavors to meld together. Turn off heat and let rest for a few minutes before serving.

8. To serve, divide soup between serving bowls and garnish with fresh herbs.

BIELER'S BROTH
(Samantha's version)

Time:

20 minutes

Serves:

1-2

Ingredients:

2 medium zucchini, chopped

1 stalk celery, chopped

1 large handful fresh or frozen green beans, chopped

2 cups water

1 generous handful fresh cilantro

Directions:

1. Place all ingredients in a pot and bring to a boil. Lower the heat and cover the pot. Continue to cook for about 15 minutes until the vegetables are tender.

2. Puree soup in a blender for 1-2 minutes and enjoy warm.

Note:

You can use Bieler's Broth as a vegetarian soup base. Just add salt and black pepper to taste.

Snacks

SWEET LASSI
(Samantha & Keith)

Time:

5 minutes

Serves:

1-2

Ingredients:

½ cup plain yogurt

1½ cups water

2 teaspoons raw honey or other sweetener

¼ teaspoon cardamom

Directions:

1. Mix all the ingredients.

2. Put in a blender until smooth.

DIGESTIVE LASSI
(Samantha & Keith)

Time:

5 minutes

Serves:

1-2

Ingredients:

½ cup plain yogurt

1½ cups water

½ teaspoon cumin

¼ teaspoon salt

3 to 4 mint leaves, or several cilantro leaves

Directions:

1. Mix all the ingredients in a blender.

2. Blend until smooth.

RICE CAKES AND AVOCADO
(Samantha & Keith)

Time:

3-5 minutes

Serves:

1-2

Ingredients:

1 avocado

2-3 rice cakes

1 pinch of salt

1 lemon

Directions:

1. For more deliciousness, toast the rice cakes on low heat.

2. Mash the avocado and add lemon and salt to taste.

SPRING DIP
(mixed sources)

Time:

10 minutes

Serves:

1-2 (makes one small bowl)

Ingredients:

½ cup peas, either fresh or frozen (defrosted)

1 avocado cubed

juice of ½ lemon or 1 lime

¼ cup finely chopped parsley and/or cilantro

2-3 fresh sprigs of mint leaves

½ teaspoon olive oil

⅓ teaspoon sea salt

Directions:

1. First rinse the peas with warm water, letting them defrost for half an hour. They don't need to be cooked but the dip is way too cold if you use totally frozen peas!

2. Drain and add lemon or lime juice, olive oil and salt.

3. Add finely chopped parsley and/or cilantro, and mint to the other ingredients and put in a food processor. It should take 2-3 minutes for a beautifully smooth consistency to form.

4. Then slather over gluten-free toast or crackers.

VARIETY PLAN: SECOND, SPECIALTY MEALS

Let's clarify a few points: Many practitioners of meditation and yoga consider garlic and onions to be activating rather than calming, and not helpful for clear meditation experiences. From the perspective of Ayurveda, garlic is a medicinal herb with many applications for healing. We have included garlic and onions in some of the specialty recipes, but they are optional and there are alternatives for those who prefer not to use them. You will also find hot spices in a few recipes. These spices can be good for detoxing the body, but they can cause hyperacidity in certain people (especially those with an Ayurvedic Pitta Nature; see Chapter 21).

Meat eaters, please note: Our expertise is on a predominantly vegetarian diet, so we do not include recipes for chicken or fish. Whatever recipe you chose, be sure to use a substitute for dairy or gluten.

Breakfast

GOLDEN MILK
(Alexis)

Time:

   10 minutes

Serves:

2

Ingredients:

1 cup unsweetened non-dairy milk, preferably coconut or almond milk

½ cup water

1 cinnamon stick or ½ teaspoon ground cinnamon

¼ teaspoon ground cardamom

1 (1-inch) piece turmeric (peeled or unpeeled and thinly sliced), or ½ teaspoon dried turmeric

1 (½-inch) piece ginger (peeled or unpeeled and thinly sliced), or ½ teaspoon dried ginger

1 tablespoon honey (do not cook)

1 tablespoon virgin coconut oil or ghee

¼ teaspoon whole black peppercorns

Directions:

1. Whisk coconut milk, cinnamon, turmeric, ginger, coconut oil, and peppercorns in a small saucepan (if using coconut milk you will want to thin it with ½ cup water; if you are using almond milk you may not need any water). Bring to a Low boil.

2. Reduce heat and simmer until flavors have melded, about 10 minutes. Strain through a fine-mesh sieve into mugs. Add honey at the very end when milk is warm, not hot.

Note:

A great option is to add this golden milk to gluten-free oatmeal and top with nuts and dried fruit for a warming, comforting breakfast. Golden milk can be stored in an airtight container in the refrigerator and kept for 2 days. Warm before serving.

GRANOLA (Alexis)

Time:

45-60 minutes (prep 15 minutes, baking 30-45 minutes)

Serves:

15

Ingredients:

3 cups gluten-free oats

½ cup gluten-free flour

½ teaspoon salt

1 teaspoon cinnamon or more to taste

½ teaspoon cardamom

1 cup slivered/chopped nuts of choice (almonds, cashews, pecans)

½ cup dried fruit of choice (chopped dates, raisins, craisins, cherries, blueberries, apricots)

½ cup virgin coconut oil or ghee

½ cup water

¼ cup maple syrup

Directions:

1. Preheat oven to 325 degrees F. Line a large baking sheet or casserole dish with parchment paper.

2. Combine all dry ingredients in large mixing bowl.

3. Combine coconut oil, water, and maple syrup in separate bowl and pour over dry ingredients. Mix until combined and mixture is moist.

4. Pour mixture onto a baking sheet and evenly distribute (should be about one inch thick). Press down with hands.

5. Place in oven for 15 minutes, then flip in large sections using a wide spatula, being careful not to break up clumps too much.

6. Bake for an additional 10-20 minutes until desired color (golden brown) is reached.

7. Remove from oven and let cool (granola will form clusters as it cools).

8. Store in airtight container in refrigerator.

GLUTEN-FREE CREPES
(Alexis)

Time:

35 minutes (prep 15 minutes, cooking 20 minutes)

Serves:

6

Ingredients:

1 cup buckwheat flour

1½ cups dairy-free milk of choice

4 eggs

1 teaspoon salt

4 tablespoons avocado oil or melted ghee or coconut oil

2 tablespoons high heat oil of choice, for cooking

Directions:

1. Sift flour and salt together in large bowl.

2. In small bowl, whisk eggs and milk.

3. Mix all ingredients until well combined—it works best to add egg/milk mixture in slowly and whisk to remove any clumps.

4. Add 4 tablespoons of avocado oil, ghee, or coconut oil.

5. Strain through a fine mesh strainer to remove any lumps, then heat a large non-stick pan over Medium heat until warm.

6. Add a bit of high heat oil of choice (avocado or coconut oil) and swirl around to cover pan.

7. Pour a small amount of batter (about ½ cup) into the middle of the pan, then tip the pan around until the batter spreads into a thin layer and is crepe shaped. Cook for about 2-3

minutes, or until bottom is golden brown when you peek at it, then carefully flip and cook the other side for 1-2 more minutes. Turn down heat if crepe is browning too much.

8. Slip onto a plate, add filling, fold and enjoy!

9. Suggested fillings:

- Goat cheese, honey, slivered almonds, and cranberries (fresh or dry)

- Sautéed kale or chard with garlic and onion, mushrooms, nutritional yeast, and garlic sauce

- Scrambled eggs with sautéed spinach and garlic. You can replace garlic with any fresh or dried herbs such as cilantro, basil, tarragon, or parsley

- Fresh berries with honey

- Almond or cashew butter with banana and toasted walnuts

Note:

For best results make the crepe batter is made the night before and stored in refrigerator overnight. Bring out 15 minutes before cooking in order to bring to room temperature, and mix batter with a whisk. This recipe makes 6 crepes. To keep: cool and stack, then put in large Ziploc bag (2 days in refrigerator or 2 months in freezer).

GLUTEN-FREE WAFFLES
(Alexis)

Time:

25 minutes (prep 10 minutes, cooking 15 minutes)

Serves:

6

Ingredients:

2 cups gluten-free flour

½ teaspoon salt

3 teaspoons baking powder

1½ cups dairy-free milk (almond, coconut, or hazelnut milk)

2 eggs

4 tablespoons ghee, melted

Directions:

1. Preheat waffle iron.

2. In large mixing bowl combine the dry ingredients.

3. In another bowl, whisk together the 1½ cups milk and eggs; stir in butter.

4. Slowly whisk the wet mixture into the dry mixture; if necessary add additional milk until batter is slightly thicker than pancake batter.

5. Spread ½ cup onto the waffle iron and cook according to manufacturer's instructions and then remove and place on

a baking rack in a 200 degree F oven to keep warm. Tip: Do not stack. Put them in a single layer to ensure crispness. Serve immediately with desired toppings, such as fresh cherry-berry compote and more maple syrup. Store leftovers in a freezer-safe bag and reheat in the toaster for best results. Will keep in the freezer for up to a couple of months, although they're best within the first couple of weeks.

CHIA PUDDING
(Alexis)

Time:

65 minutes (5-10 minutes assembly and mixing, 1 hour to set/thicken)

Serves:

2

Ingredients:

6 tablespoons chia seeds

2 cups unsweetened coconut, almond, hazelnut, or cashew milk

½ teaspoon vanilla extract

1 tablespoon maple syrup, honey or sweetener of choice (optional)

½ teaspoon cinnamon (optional)

¼ teaspoon cardamom (optional)

blueberries, strawberries, or other fruit, for topping

nuts or seeds of choice for topping

Directions:

1. In a bowl or mason jar, mix together chia seeds, milk, maple syrup and vanilla. If you're using a mason jar, you can put the lid on and shake the mixture to combine everything.

2. Once the chia pudding mixture is well combined, let it sit for 5 minutes, give it another stir/shake to break up any clumps of chia seeds, cover and put the mixture in the fridge to set for 1-2 hours or overnight. The chia pudding should be nice and thick, not liquidy. If it's not thick, just add more chia seeds, stir and refrigerate for another 30 minutes or so.

3. You can also prep your pudding the night before and let it sit in the fridge overnight. When ready to serve, divide the mixture between two bowls, top with berries and nuts.

GLUTEN-FREE FRENCH TOAST
(Alexis)

Time:

25 minutes (prep 10 minutes, cooking 15 minutes)

Serves:

1-2

Ingredients:

2 slices gluten-free bread

1 egg, beaten

¼ cup dairy-free milk, such as coconut, hazelnut, or almond milk

1 teaspoon maple syrup

¼ teaspoon cinnamon

¼ teaspoon cardamom

¼ teaspoon salt

¼ teaspoon vanilla extract

1 tablespoon ghee for frying

Directions:

1. Combine eggs, hazelnut, coconut or almond milk, maple syrup, salt, and vanilla in a bowl. Whisk until thoroughly blended.

2. Dip slices of bread in the egg mixture. Allow both sides of the bread to soak up as much of the mixture as it will hold (like a sponge!).

3. Heat ghee on Medium-High in a large, heavy skillet and fry coated bread slices. When golden brown, flip and cook the second side until golden brown.

4. Serve with ghee, maple syrup, berries, and lemon zest.

EGG SCRAMBLE WITH AVOCADO
(Alexis)

Time:

20 minutes (prep 10 minutes, cooking 10 minutes)

Serves:

1

Ingredients:

2 eggs

½ cup spinach

¼ avocado

½ medium tomato, diced

1 clove garlic, finely minced (optional, see note)

1 small shallot, finely diced (optional, see note)

½ cup red pepper or any seasonal vegetables, chopped

Salt, pepper, and fresh herbs (basil, cilantro, etc.) to taste

Directions:

1. Heat a medium pan, coat with ½ teaspoon olive oil.

2. Sauté garlic and shallot until golden brown.

3. Add the red pepper and other vegetables, cook until tender.

4. Add tomato, spinach, and eggs.

5. Cook until eggs are set.

6. Transfer to serving plate and slice ¼ avocado over top.

Note:

If you are avoiding garlic and/or onion, omit the garlic and shallot, and simply cook egg in oil of choice and add desired fresh or dried herbs (basil, parsley, cilantro, fennel).

CRISPY HAYSTACKS
(Alexis, inspired by Minimalist Baker)

Time:

55 minutes (prep 20 minutes, cooking 35 minutes)

Serves:

6

Ingredients:

½ cup loosely packed finely grated russet potato, washed and scrubbed (1 small potato yields ½ cup)

½ cup small zucchini, grated

1 small shallot, very thinly sliced (optional)

¼ cup fresh chopped parsley (or other herb of choice)

¼ cup corn (preferably fresh; if canned, very well drained)

2 tablespoons coconut oil

½ tablespoon cornstarch or arrowroot starch (for binding)

¼ teaspoon each sea salt and black pepper (plus more to taste)

Directions:

1. Preheat oven to 375 degrees F and generously grease a muffin tin with oil of choice.

2. I do not peel my potatoes or yams (that is where a lot of the nutrients are) but it is by preference.

3. Add finely grated potatoes and zucchini to a large mixing bowl with shallot, parsley, corn, melted coconut oil, cornstarch, salt and pepper. Stir to thoroughly combine.

4. Divide mixture evenly among 6 muffin tins, filling each tin with about 1/4 cup of the potato mixture. Press down gently to form. Sprinkle the tops with a pinch more salt and pepper and bake for 15 minutes.

5. After 15 minutes, increase oven temperature to 425 degrees F and bake for 10-12 minutes more, or until the tops appear golden brown and the edges are dark golden brown.

6. Remove from oven and let rest for 5 minutes, then loosen the sides with a butter knife and gently lift out with a fork. Serve immediately or add sauce of choice. (These are especially great with a poached egg.)

7. Best when fresh. To freeze, arrange baked haystacks in a single layer on a baking sheet and freeze until firm. Then store in a freezer-safe container up to 3-4 weeks.

8. Reheat in a 350 degree F oven until completely warmed through.

Lunch and Dinner

MACRO LUNCH BOWL

(Alexis)

Time:

60-75 minutes (prep 30-45 minutes, cooking 20 minutes, 5 minutes assembly)

Serves:

1

Ingredients:

4 teaspoons olive oil

¼ white onion, diced (optional)

1-2 cloves garlic, finely chopped (optional)

½ cup broccoli or cauliflower, cut into bite-sized pieces and roasted

½ cup sweet potato, cut into bite-sized pieces and roasted

½ cup Swiss chard, kale, or spinach, roughly chopped

1 egg, pasture raised if possible, hard boiled

¼ medium avocado

½ lemon

2 teaspoons gluten-free liquid aminos (such as Bragg Liquid Aminos)

1 teaspoon sesame seeds

¾ teaspoon turmeric

salt and pepper to taste

1 slice of gluten-free bread, toasted or ½ cup prepared quinoa or other gluten-free grain (rice, millet, couscous)

Directions:

1. Heat oven to 400 degrees F. Chop broccoli, cauliflower, and sweet potato into large bite-sized pieces. Keep separated and put into individual small mixing bowls. Add 1 teaspoon olive oil to each, with ½ teaspoon of turmeric, and salt and pepper to taste. Mix to evenly coat.

2. Spread on lined baking sheet in a single layer, keep each vegetable group separate. Roast for 10-15 minutes or until tender.

3. Bring a small pot of water to a boil over High heat. Reduce heat to Low, then add egg and cook 4-5 minutes. Drain off water and cool in ice water, then peel. If you want a harder egg, boil 1-2 minutes longer.

4. When using gluten-free grain, prepare following package instructions, or toast bread.

5. Heat the oil in a skillet on Medium temperature. Sauté the garlic and onion for 2 minutes until soft. Skip this step if you are avoiding onion and/or garlic.

6. Add the leafy greens and liquid aminos, cooking for another minute. Remove from heat.

7. Assemble ingredients in your favorite bowl, using the gluten-free grain as a base, then leafy greens, then roasted vegetables, and egg.

8. Squeeze lemon juice and sprinkle with sesame seeds. Season to taste with salt and pepper.

VEGAN GREEN BEAN CASSEROLE
(Alexis)

Time:

60 minutes (prep 30 minutes, cooking 30 minutes)

Serves:

4

*If you do not want to use garlic, onion, or shallots then use 20-25 mushrooms, and follow recipe accordingly. For a topper, use fresh herbs. (Parsley would be a nice addition to this dish.)

Ingredients:

2 shallots, thinly sliced (optional)
1 medium yellow onion, thinly sliced (optional)
1 tablespoon olive oil or ghee
6 tablespoons high heat oil
2 cups turnips or parsnips, cubed and steamed
10-12 mushrooms, sliced
1 lb. fresh green beans, cut into 1-inch pieces and steamed
3 cloves garlic, minced (optional)

½ cup nutritional yeast

½ cup water

1½ teaspoons fine sea salt

Pepper to taste

Directions:

1. Preheat oven to 350 degrees F.

2. If including onion and garlic: In a large pan over Medium heat add the olive oil or ghee, onion, and garlic, until translucent. Add the mushrooms and cook until liquid is released, about 6 minutes.

3. Prepare turnips or parsnips and green beans by cutting and steaming (keep separate) for 6-8 minutes until you can pierce turnips or parsnips with a fork, and green beans are bright green and tender but still have a bit of crunch. Set the green beans aside.

4. Add the turnips or parsnips, water, nutritional yeast, salt, pepper, and half of the mushroom, onion, and garlic mixture with any liquid to blender. Blend until smooth and creamy, add salt, pepper, or nutritional yeast for desired taste.

5. Add remaining ½ mushroom, onion, and garlic mixture to green beans. Mix mushroom and green bean mixture with sauce.

6. Transfer to a greased 8x8 casserole dish. Bake for 25-30 minutes or until bubbling.

7. While casserole is bubbling add 6 tablespoons high heat oil to small pan over High heat. Add shallots to oil when hot, and fry until golden brown. Remove and place on a paper towel lined plate.

8. Remove casserole from oven and allow to cool 5 minutes. Top with crispy shallots and enjoy!

ZUCCHINI GRATIN
(Alexis inspired by the Minimalist Baker)

Time:
60 minutes (prep 30 minutes, baking 30 minutes)

Serves:

6

*This recipe is not recommended for those avoiding garlic and/or onion

Ingredients:
For the Vegan Creamy Cheese Sauce:

1 cup raw cashews

¾ cup nutritional yeast

1 teaspoon salt

¼ teaspoon garlic powder

¼ teaspoon onion powder

For the Gratin:

2 medium zucchini squash, sliced into thin rounds (you can use green or yellow, or mix for visual beauty)

¾ medium yellow or white onion (cut into thin rings)

1 teaspoon each sea salt and black pepper

3 tablespoons olive oil

handful of roughly chopped parsley

Directions:

1. Prepare vegan cheese sauce by combining all ingredients together in a blender, and slowly add water until mixture is a creamy consistency.

2. In a 10-inch cast iron or oven-safe skillet, sauté onion in 1 tablespoon olive oil over Medium-Low heat until soft (about 10 minutes), seasoning with a pinch of salt and black pepper. Spread slightly cooled onions around in the bottom of the skillet to create an even base. Pour cheese sauce over the top of the onions.

3. Preheat oven to 400 degrees F.

4. Slice squash into very thin slices, about 1/8-inch thick. Use a mandoline slicer if you have one, or just a sharp knife.

5. Top the onion and cheese layers with squash, layering green and yellow as you go (if you did two colors). It doesn't have

to be perfect. Just start on the outside and work your way in, keeping them in line as much as possible.

6. Top with gluten-free breadcrumbs.

7. Bake at 400 degrees F for 30 minutes. Let rest for a few minutes before serving. Sprinkle with roughly chopped parsley.

8. Reheats well in the oven.

GLUTEN-FREE ENCHILADAS
(Alexis)

Time:
60-65 minutes (prep 35 minutes, baking 25-30 minutes)
* soak beans overnight

Serves:
2-3

Ingredients:
Premade gluten-free flour tortillas

Burrito Filling:
1½ cup salsa or tomatoes if avoiding garlic and/or onion
½ cup plain, cooked brown rice
1 tablespoon olive oil
½ red onion, diced fine (optional)
1 clove garlic, minced (optional)

5 mushrooms, chopped

1 red, orange or yellow pepper

1 cup spinach, lightly sautéed

2 teaspoon cumin

1 tablespoon fresh cilantro, chopped (optional)

1 cup beans (black, great northern, or pinto)

½ cup corn

salt and pepper, to taste

¼ cup nutritional yeast

Optional toppings:

fresh cilantro, chopped

fresh tomatoes, diced

avocado, avocado crema (see below), or guacamole (also see below)

Directions:

1. Soak beans overnight OR put beans in a pot, cover with water, bring them to a boil. Boil for two minutes then remove from heat. Let sit for 1 hour in water. Drain off water. Put beans in pot and cover with fresh water. Bring to a boil and cook until done.

2. Preheat oven to 350 degrees F. Lightly oil a large casserole dish. Spread 1 cup of salsa or tomatoes on the bottom of the pan.

3. Prepare long-grain brown rice, use 2/3 cup water to 1/2 cup rice. For short-grain rice, use 3/4 cup water. Bring rice, water,

and salt (1/8 teaspoon) to a boil. Cover, and reduce to a slow, steady simmer for 30-40 minutes. Let the cooked rice sit for 10 minutes, covered, to absorb maximum moisture; then remove the lid, and fluff the grains with a fork.

4. Heat one tablespoon of oil in a large sauté pan over Medium-High heat. Add onion and garlic and sauté until translucent. Add mushrooms, peppers or other vegetables of choice. Sauté for 5 minutes or until the vegetables are softer and starting to brown. Add spinach and mix in.

5. Add the cumin, cilantro, beans, corn and salsa, stirring while cooking until warmed. Taste and add salt and pepper if needed. Stir the cooked rice into vegetable mixture.

6. Spoon a row of the vegetable filling in a line down the center of one gluten-free flour tortilla. There are two ways to prepare the burrito from here: you can either roll up opposite ends of the tortilla (the two sides at the end of the row of filling) and then roll the tortilla up, starting with one of the remaining sides and tucking it around the filling, then roll the burrito around itself tightly OR simply roll the tortilla up around the filling.

7. Lay the burrito seam-down in the salsa-covered pan. Continue with remaining tortillas. Spread ½ cup additional salsa or tomatoes on top of the tortillas and bake uncovered for 25 minutes. If at any time the tortillas start to brown too much, cover the pan with foil and continue baking.

8. Remove from oven and let cool for 5 minutes. Sprinkle nutritional yeast and desired toppings on top of enchiladas and serve.

SAVORY POLENTA CAKES
(Alexis)

Time:

105 minutes (prep 90 minutes, cooking 15 minutes)

Serves:

4-6

Ingredients:

4 cups water

1 cup finely ground cornmeal

1 teaspoon sea salt

1 tablespoon olive oil

1 tablespoon chopped rosemary, oregano, or thyme (optional)

Directions:

1. In a large saucepan, bring water to a rolling boil. Add salt and reduce to a simmer. Gradually whisk in the cornmeal. Once all cornmeal is added, continually stir with a wooden spoon. Reduce heat to Low and continue to cook until mixture thickens, stirring often. Add desired herbs.

2. Once the polenta has thickened (approximately 10-15 minutes), check for seasoning and add salt if necessary. Then pour the mixture into a small glass casserole dish. Add a layer of parchment paper on top and smooth it down directly on the polenta. Place into the refrigerator for approximately 30 minutes to set. (You can place in freezer to speed the process.)

3. When you are ready to make the polenta cakes, use a round cookie cutter or a glass to make 6 polenta circles or "cakes."

4. Place a sauté pan over Medium heat and add approximately 1 tablespoon of extra virgin olive oil. When the oil is hot, place the polenta circles into the pan. Cook until a golden-ish crust has formed on both sides, turning as little as possible. OR coat cakes in gluten-free breadcrumbs and place on parchment-lined baking sheet and bake at 400 degrees F for 10-15 minutes, flipping halfway if necessary, until golden brown. Delicious topped with sautéed veggies and tomato confit! (see recipe)

FAUX AHI TUNA AND AVOCADO SALSA
(Alexis)

Time:

30 minutes

Serves:

4-6

Ingredients:

3 large tomatoes, blanched, peeled, seeded, and sliced into one-inch cubes (this is faux ahi tuna)

3 large avocados, cubed

1 tablespoon of sesame seeds

1 teaspoon olive oil

1 teaspoon grated ginger

salt and pepper to taste

Directions:

1. Make an X on the bottom of your tomatoes and throw them into a pot of boiling water for no more than a minute. Fish them out with a slotted spoon, plunge them into a bowl of cold water (or an ice bath), lift them directly back out, and peel back the skin with a knife or your fingers. It will slip off like a charm.

2. Cut tomatoes into lengthwise slices and remove seedy flesh, use remaining flesh and cut into cubes.

3. Mix with the rest of the ingredients in large mixing bowl to combine. Enjoy!

AVOCADO SUSHI
(Alexis)

Time:

60 minutes (prep 30 minutes, 30 minutes assembly)

Serves:

4-6

Ingredients:

4 nori (seaweed) sheets

1 avocado

2 cups sushi rice

2 cups water

⅓ cup rice vinegar

1 teaspoon salt

black and white sesame seeds, optional

bamboo rolling mat

Directions:

1. Cook sushi rice in boiling water or rice cooker. When cooked, add rice vinegar and salt, set aside and let cool.

2. Cut avocado into thin slices.

3. Cover bamboo mat in cellophane or with a Ziploc bag.

4. Lay a sheet of nori, shiny side down, on the mat.

5. With wet fingers (dip in rice vinegar or water), spread ½ cup rice on nori.

6. Sprinkle with sesame seeds, and then gently flip over.

7. Place ¼of the avocados in the center of the sheet. Roll sushi, pressing tightly on the mat for a firm roll.

8. Slice into 6 pieces. If knife gets sticky, dip in rice vinegar or water. Repeat with remaining nori sheets and vegetables.

9. Serve with amino acids and/or wasabi and/or pickled ginger.

TWICE BAKED SWEET POTATOES WITH COCONUT OIL AND CINNAMON
(Alexis)

Time:

105 minutes (prep 30 minutes, baking 75 minutes)

Serves:

4

Ingredients:

2 large sweet potatoes, scrubbed

2 tablespoons coconut oil, melted

2 teaspoons ground cinnamon

¼ cup almond, hazelnut, or coconut milk

½ cup roasted cashews or hazelnuts, roughly chopped

sea salt and pepper to taste

Directions:

1. Preheat the oven to 350 degrees F.

2. Pierce each sweet potato a few times with a fork, then place them on a baking sheet and bake until tender, 45 to 60 minutes.

3. When the sweet potatoes are tender, let them cool until they are easily handled. Cut each sweet potato in half lengthwise and scoop out all but a ¼-inch wall of the flesh.

4. Add the scooped sweet potato flesh to a large mixing bowl with coconut oil, cinnamon, nut milk, sea salt and pepper. Mix well until smooth and the texture of whipped potatoes.

5. Spoon the filling into each of the sweet potato halves and place them back on the baking sheet. Bake until the tops of the sweet potatoes start to brown, about 20 minutes.

6. Serve topped with either roasted cashews, sunflower seeds, hazelnuts, or fresh herbs such as basil.

POLENTA CUP
(Alexis)

Time:

  60 minutes (prep 45 minutes, baking 15 minutes)

Serves:

  4

Ingredients:

  2 cups water
  ½ teaspoon salt
  ½ cup yellow cornmeal
  ½ teaspoon minced fresh thyme or ¼ teaspoon dried thyme
  ¼ teaspoon pepper

2 plum tomatoes, finely chopped

2 cups spinach, sautéed with diced onion (onion optional)

2 tablespoons olive or coconut oil

¼ cup crumbled goat cheese

2 tablespoons chopped fresh basil

1 garlic clove, minced (optional)

1 egg (optional)

Directions:

1. In a large heavy saucepan, bring water and salt to a boil.
   Reduce heat to a gentle boil; slowly whisk in cornmeal. Cook
   and stir with a wooden spoon for 10-15 minutes or until
   polenta is thickened and pulls away cleanly from the sides of
   the pan. Remove from the heat; stir in thyme and pepper.

2. Brush muffin tins with olive or coconut oil. Spoon heaping
   tablespoonfuls into muffin cups. Using the back of a spoon,
   make an indentation in the center of each. Cover and chill
   until set. Meanwhile, in a small bowl, combine the tomatoes,
   onion, spinach, basil, and garlic.

3. To sauté spinach, heat 1 teaspoon olive oil in small pan over
   medium heat. Add the onion if using. Cook until translucent.
   Add spinach and cook until wilted, about 1 minute.

4. Unmold polenta cups and place on an ungreased baking
   sheet. Top each with 1 heaping tablespoon of tomato mixture
   and, if desired, crack a raw egg in and bake until set. Broil 4
   inches from the heat for 5-7 minutes or until heated through.

Top with goat cheese, tomato confit, garlic sauce, sautéed spinach, or any other desired topping and enjoy!

ROASTED FENNEL WITH PRESERVED LEMONS AND GLUTEN-FREE BREADCRUMBS
(Alexis)

Time:

30 minutes (prep 15 minutes, baking 15 minutes)

Serves:

4-6

Ingredients:

2-3 fennel bulbs

1 teaspoon from a jar of preserved lemons

2 tablespoons olive oil

½ cup gluten-free bread crumbs

1 teaspoon salt

cracked pepper to taste

Directions:

1. Preheat oven to 425 F degrees.

2. Prepare the fennel by removing green stalks about 1 inch above the fennel bulb. Place one hand toward the top of the fennel bulb to steady it. Using a sharp knife, slice off the root end of the bulb. Cut each fennel lengthwise into two pieces. Remove the tough core from the fennel halves by cutting

a wedge-shape piece from the top of the tough core to the bottom. Discard this core. Slice the fennel halves in quarters and then lengthwise into wedges.

3. Remove a quarter of lemon from the jar of preserved lemons and rinse under cold water. If you skip this step, the salt on the lemon will be overpowering. Pat the lemon dry and separate the peel from the flesh using a sharp knife. Finely mince the rind.

4. In a large bowl, mix the fennel, preserved lemons, olive oil, salt, and pepper. Mix until evenly coated.

5. Evenly distribute fennel in single layer on baking sheet lined with parchment paper.

6. Roast for 12-15 minutes or until fennel starts to darken on the bottom.

7. Place in baking dish and sprinkle with gluten-free breadcrumbs.

VIETNAMESE SPRING ROLL WITH DIPPING SAUCE
(Alexis)

Time:
   30-45 minutes
Serves:
   4

Ingredients:

½ red pepper, julienned and steamed until you can pierce with a fork

1 large carrot, julienned and steamed until you can pierce with a fork

½ cup baby spinach, lightly sautéed

3 green onions, thinly sliced on a diagonal (optional)

6 rice papers

1 package rice vermicelli (very thin rice noodles), cooked

sesame seeds

Dipping Sauce

1 tablespoon Bragg Liquid Aminos or coconut aminos

1 tablespoon toasted sesame oil

1 tablespoon maple syrup

2-3 tablespoons water to thin

Directions:

1. Prepare all your ingredients. Julienne vegetables by cutting into long thin strips 1/8 inches by 2 inches.

2. Prep your area: Find a nice clean space of counter to work on, fill a large bowl or pie plate with HOT water, and gather all of your prepped veggies and sesame seeds.

3. Rice paper is delicate and only needs a quick dip in warm water until it is soft and flexible (about 3 seconds). Do not "soak" the rice paper for too long because it will break

down quickly, making it more difficult to roll. Rotate the immersed rice paper in the bowl of water. Remove from water; it will still be slightly firm. Gently shake excess water from the rice paper, lay it flat on preparation surface.

4. Let it sit for a further 30 seconds to absorb any excess water.

5. Sprinkle a portion of sesame seeds in the center of the wrap.

6. Lay the julienned vegetables down in the middle of the wrap. Use approximately ¼ of each ingredient per wrap (use a little more or a little less depending on how many wraps you want to make and how big you'd like them). Try to keep the fillings laid neatly, making sure to leave ample room on each side to easily fold the wrap.

7. Lift the side of the rice paper that's closest to you, and gently pull it forward (away from you) over the fillings. Hold the wrap firmly while you fold in each end of the wrap. Continue rolling to seal the seam.

8. Dipping Sauce:

   - Combine all ingredients in a bowl and whisk vigorously OR combine all ingredients in food processor and pulse.

   - Store extra sauce in the fridge. It may thicken when refrigerated, but you can soften it back to a liquid by placing the container in hot water.

Soups

TUSCAN WHITE BEAN AND POTATO SOUP WITH ROSEMARY
(Alexis)

Time:

40-55 minutes (prep 10-15 minutes, cooking 30-40 minutes)

*soak beans overnight OR put beans in a pot, cover with water, bring them to a boil. Boil for two minutes then remove from heat. Let sit for 1 hour in the water. Then drain off water. Put beans in pot and cover with fresh water. Bring to a boil and cook until done.

Serves:

4-6

Ingredients:

2 tablespoons olive oil

1 white onion and/or 1½ cup celery, diced

3 cloves garlic, minced (optional)

½ teaspoon red chili flakes (optional)

2 sprigs rosemary, chopped fine

3 cups cannellini or navy beans

1½ cup water or more to taste, depending on desired texture

10 small potatoes, halved or quartered

salt and pepper to taste

Directions:

1. In a large pot over Medium heat, add olive oil, white onion, red chili flakes (optional), garlic (optional), and rosemary. Sauté 5 minutes until onions are golden.

2. Add in the cannellini beans and water, bring to a simmer.

3. Add potatoes and let cook for 10 minutes. Salt and pepper to taste.

4. To have a creamy soup, remove half and blend in blender, add back to soup.

5. Serve with a dollop of yogurt, fresh parsley, and sunflower seeds.

Note:

If you omit garlic, you can add more rosemary to taste for flavor. If you are avoiding onion, use sautéed celery.

TORTILLA SOUP
(Alexis)

Time:

40-55 minutes (prep 10-15 minutes, cooking 30-40 minutes)

Serves:

4-6

Ingredients:

2 tablespoons olive oil

2 white onions

3 yellow, red, or orange peppers, chopped

2 cloves garlic, minced (optional)

2 tablespoons ground cumin

1 cup crushed tomatoes

4 cups vegetable broth

salt and pepper to taste

1 cup whole kernel corn

gluten-free tortilla chips

1 avocado, peeled, pitted and diced

Directions:

1. Heat the oil in a large pot over Medium heat. Stir in garlic, onion, and cumin, and cook 5 minutes.

2. Add the peppers, and cook an additional 5 minutes.

3. Mix in the tomatoes. Pour in the broth, and season with salt and pepper. Bring to a boil, reduce heat to Low, and simmer 30 minutes.

4. For a smooth soup, blend.

5. Mix corn into the soup, and continue cooking 5 minutes. Serve in bowls over equal amounts of tortilla chips. Top with avocado and cilantro.

INDIAN DAHL SOUP
(Danielle Wallace, see craftydutchgirl.com)

Time:

3-8 hours depending on how it is cooked (prep 10 minutes, cooking 3-8 hours)

Serves:

6

Ingredients:

1 cup red lentils

1 cup mung dhal (yellow lentils)

6 cups water

2 cubes vegetable bouillon

3 cups any vegetable (zucchini, carrots, chard, kale, broccoli, celery)

3 tablespoons butter

1 teaspoon salt

½ teaspoon garlic powder

½ teaspoon mustard seeds

½ teaspoon cumin

½ teaspoon turmeric

½ teaspoon cinnamon

Directions:

1. Turn the crock pot on Low and cook between 6-8 hours. Turn it on High if you only have 3-5 hours. Clean lentils under cold running water. Add water, lentils, vegetables and

the 2 bouillon cubes to the crock pot and cook for 3-8 hours, depending on the setting.

2. Melt the butter in a sauce pan. Add all the spices and mix with a wooden spoon. Add the spices to the soup. Blend with a stick blender and taste.

3. Serve with Basmati rice, yogurt, and raisins.

Note:

This wonderful Indian Dahl Soup can serve as a full meal.

Snacks, Sauces, and Desserts

KALE CHIP NACHOS
(Alexis)

Time:

80-100 minutes (prep 30 minutes, baking 40-70 minutes, less time with pressure cooker)

*soak beans overnight.

Serves:

2-4

Ingredients:

2-3 heads curly kale, washed and thoroughly dried

2 tablespoons olive oil

Sea salt and pepper

½ teaspoon garlic powder (optional)

¼ teaspoon cumin

¼ teaspoon ground red pepper (optional)

¼ teaspoon chili powder (optional)

1 cup black beans, cooked

½ cup salsa

½ small chopped onion (optional)

3 chives or chopped green onion (optional)

handful of cilantro leaves

⅓ cup goat cheese or nutritional yeast

Directions:

1. Bring the beans to a boil. Remove any scum that forms. Boil for 10 minutes, cover and turn the heat down to Low. Simmer until the beans still hold their shape but are tender, about 40 minutes to 1 hour depending on the age of the beans.

2. If you want to use a pressure cooker, then combine 1 cup of beans, 2½ cups of water, 1 tablespoon olive oil, and 1 teaspoon of salt, making sure it's no more than halfway full. Secure the lid. Make sure the pressure regulator valve is closed. Cook for approximately 20 minutes. Double-check

the manual that came with your pressure cooker for more exact cooking times.

3. Preheat the oven to 275 degrees F.

4. Remove the ribs from the kale and cut into 1½-inch pieces. Lay on a baking sheet and toss with the olive oil and salt. Bake until crisp, turning the leaves halfway through, about 20 minutes.

5. Heat oven to 350 degrees F.

6. Mix the black beans with some of the salsa in a small bowl and set aside.

7. Spread the kale chips on a baking sheet and begin the layering process. Add bean and salsa mixture, onions, chives, and goat cheese/nutritional yeast.

8. Pop these babies in the oven and bake 8-10 minutes. Eat with a fork :-)

VEGAN AVOCADO CREMA
(Alexis)

Time:

10 minutes

Serves:

2-4

Ingredients:

1 ripe avocado

3 tablespoons lime juice

1-2 tablespoons water, depending on desired thickness

½ teaspoon sea salt

¼ cup fresh cilantro leaves

Directions:

1. Combine all ingredients.

2. Put in a blender and blend until smooth.

GUACAMOLE
(Alexis)

Time:

30 minutes

Serves:

4-6

Ingredients:

4 medium ripe avocados, halved and cubed

2 medium diced tomatoes (optional)

½ red onion, diced (optional)

½ cup cilantro, chopped

1 large clove of garlic, minced (optional)

3 limes juiced

1 teaspoon cumin

1 teaspoon salt

Directions:

1. Combine all ingredients.

2. Mash with large fork or use a hand blender until desired smoothness is reached.

ROASTED BEET AND WHITE BEAN HUMMUS
(Alexis)

Time:

1 hour (including roasting beet and garlic)

Serving:

4

Ingredients

½ large beet, roasted and peeled

½ cup white beans, prepared

1 teaspoon tahini (optional)

2 large minced garlic cloves (optional)

½ cup packed basil (optional but adds flavor if omitting garlic)

1 lemon, juiced (more if omitting garlic)

⅓ cup olive oil

1 teaspoon salt (to taste)

pepper to taste

Directions:

1. Preheat oven to 400 degrees F.

2. Wash beet well and wrap (along with garlic clove, optional) in aluminum foil.

3. Bake for 45 minutes or until beet is tender when poked with a knife.

4. Remove skin from the beet and the garlic (optional).

5. Place all the ingredients in a food processor and puree until smooth.

6. Delicious spread on toast or as a dip accompanying gluten-free crackers and veggies.

VEGAN ROASTED RED PEPPER SAUCE
(Alexis)

Time:

15 minutes

*soak cashews 4 hours

Serves:

4

Ingredients:

2 large pieces of roasted red pepper from a jar

¾ cup cashews, soaked in water for at least 4 hours and drained

4 slices of jalapeno peppers (optional)

½ cup of water or more depending on desired consistency

1 teaspoon apple cider vinegar

1 teaspoon salt

pepper to taste

Directions:

1. Combine all ingredients in blender.

2. Blend until smooth.

Note:

If avoiding spicy foods, omit jalapeno peppers and substitute ½ cup packed cilantro.

TOMATO CONFIT
(Alexis)

Time:

1-1½ hours baking

Serves:

4

Ingredients:

2 cups cherry tomatoes

¼ cup olive oil

1½ teaspoons sea salt

1 teaspoon black pepper

10 peeled garlic cloves (optional)

8 large thyme sprigs or a pinch of saffron

Directions:

1. Preheat oven to 275 degrees F. Spread tomatoes onto a large rimmed baking sheet. Add oil, salt, pepper, and garlic; toss gently to coat. Tuck thyme sprigs into mixture. Bake at 275 degrees F until tomatoes are wilted but not all have burst, 1½ to 2 hours.

2. Cool tomato mixture to room temperature and discard thyme. Store tomatoes with oil and accumulated pan juices in an airtight container in refrigerator up to 2 weeks, or freeze up to 2 months.

CRISPY CHICKPEAS
(Alexis)

Time:

55-65 minutes (prep 5 minutes, 30-40 minutes cooking, baking 20 minutes)

*soak chickpeas overnight

Serves:

2-4

Ingredients:

2 cups chickpeas, cooked

2 tablespoons olive oil

¼ teaspoon smoked paprika

½ teaspoon sea salt

cracked pepper to taste

Directions:

1. Cook chickpeas for 30-40 minutes

2. OR if you did not soak overnight, put chickpeas in a pot, cover with water, bring them to a boil for two minutes, then remove from heat. Let sit for 1 hour in water. Then drain off water. Put chickpeas in pot and cover with water. Bring to a boil and cook until done.

3. Preheat oven to 425 degrees F.

4. In a large bowl, add additional ingredients to chickpeas and mix to evenly coat.

5. Spread chickpeas on baking sheet in a single layer.

6. Bake for 10 minutes, then shake tray to turn chickpeas.

7. Bake until crispy, approximately 20 minutes.

BABAGANOUSH
(Alexis)

Time:

60 minutes (prep 15 minutes, charring/baking 45 minutes)

Serves:

2-4

Ingredients:

2 small-to-medium eggplants

2 medium cloves of garlic (optional), pressed or minced

2 tablespoons lemon juice, more if necessary

¼ cup tahini

⅓ cup extra-virgin olive oil

2 tablespoons chopped fresh flat-leaf parsley

¾ teaspoon salt, to taste

¼ teaspoon ground cumin

Pinch of smoked paprika, for garnish

Directions:

1. Char the eggplants over gas stovetop burner on all sides or under the broiler in oven.

2. Place eggplants on baking sheet and cover with aluminum foil. Roast in oven at 400 degrees F for 30-40 minutes or until you can pierce with a fork.

3. Place the eggplants in a bowl, cover and let rest to cool.

4. Once you place the charred eggplant in a covered bowl it sweats and releases liquid. This liquid can be used to thin out babaganoush to desired consistency.

5. Prepare and combine other ingredients in a blender or food processor.

6. Remove skin (charred blackened layer) of eggplant and stem. Place meat of eggplant in blender or food processor with other ingredients, and add half of the liquid from the eggplant, more if necessary.

7. Serving suggestions: warmed or toasted pita wedges.

BAKED ZUCCHINI CHIPS
(adapted from A Spicy Perspective)

Time:

2 hours and 20 minutes (prep 20 minutes, cooking 2 hours)

Serving:

8

Ingredients:

4 large zucchini, evenly sliced 1/8 inch thick

2 tablespoons olive oil

Salt

½ teaspoon hot smoked paprika, optional

½ teaspoon cumin, optional

Directions:

1. Slice the zucchini. (Using a mandoline helps keep the slices consistent.) Lay the zucchini slices on paper towels in a single layer. Cover with more paper towels and set a baking sheet on top of the zucchini slices. Press down on the baking sheet, applying slight pressure, to help squeeze out some of the moisture.

2. Preheat oven to 235 degrees F. Line several baking sheets with parchment paper. Brush the parchment paper lightly with olive oil.

3. Lay the zucchini slices in a single layer on the parchment paper. Fit as many on each sheet as possible. Then lightly brush the top of the zucchini with olive oil and sprinkle with salt. For extra flavor, you can also sprinkle with a little cumin and smoked paprika.

4. Bake for 1½ -2 hours until crisp and golden. If some zucchini chips are still a little flimsy or damp, remove the crisp chips and place the damp chips back in the oven for a few minutes. Allow the zucchini chips to cool on the paper towels to absorb extra oil. Store in an airtight container.

GLUTEN-FREE VEGAN CORNBREAD
(Alexis)

Time:

45 minutes (prep 15 minutes, baking 30 minutes)

Serves:

8-10

Ingredients:

2 ½ cups unsweetened almond milk (or other nut or plant-based milk)

2 tablespoons apple cider vinegar

½ cup coconut oil (olive or vegetable oil)

8 tablespoons maple syrup (one tablespoon per serving)

Pinch of salt

1¾ cups fine cornmeal

1½ cups gluten-free flour blend

6 teaspoons baking powder

½ teaspoon baking soda

Directions:

1. Preheat the oven to 350 degrees F.

2. Measure out the milk and stir in the vinegar - set aside for at least 5 minutes to curdle.

3. Place the coconut oil in a large bowl and melt over a saucepan of boiling water (skip this step if using any other oil).

4. Add the maple syrup, salt, and cornmeal.

5. Sift in the flour, baking powder, and baking soda.

6. Add the milk and vinegar mixture. Mix well, adding extra milk or water if too dry.

7. Transfer the mixture to a square baking tin (I used a 9inch/23cm square baking tin) lined with greased baking paper and bake in the oven for around 30 minutes, until an inserted toothpick or knife comes out clean.

8. Leave to cool slightly before cutting.

9. Keeps well covered in the fridge for a few days, and freezes well too. Delicious reheated in the toaster.

GLUTEN-FREE ZUCCHINI CAKE
(Alexis)

Time:

65-80 minutes (prep 20 minutes, baking 45-60 minutes)

Serves:

8-10

Ingredients:

1½ cups grated zucchini

1 teaspoon vanilla

1 teaspoon baking powder

1 teaspoon baking soda

¼ cup olive or melted coconut oil

1 cup unsweetened applesauce

2 eggs

½ teaspoon cinnamon

1½ cups gluten-free flour blend

¾ cup almond meal (ground from raw almonds)

¼ cup gluten-free oats

1 teaspoon salt

Directions:

1. Preheat oven to 300 degrees F. Butter and flour an 8x8 pan with dairy-free butter and gluten-free flour.

2. In a large mixing bowl, whisk together oil, applesauce, eggs, and zucchini.

3. Add vanilla, baking soda, baking powder, and cinnamon. Lastly add almond meal, gluten-free flour blend, and gluten-free oats and whisk again to combine. The batter should be slightly thick but very easy to pour.

4. Pour batter into your pan and bake for 45 minutes to 1 hour, until an inserted toothpick comes out clean, and the edges of the cake are golden brown.

5. The cake should keep covered in the fridge for several days, or in the freezer for several weeks. However, it's best when eaten fresh!

6. If refrigerating, set out for 10-15 minutes before serving so it warms a bit and becomes more tender.

MAPLE ALMOND COOKIES
(Alexis)

Time:

22 minutes (prep 10 minutes, baking 10-12 minutes)

Serves:

10-12

Ingredients:

2 cups finely ground almond flour

½ teaspoon baking powder

⅓ cup maple syrup

1 teaspoon vanilla

Directions:

1. Preheat oven to 350 degrees F.

2. Combine and mix almond flour and baking powder.

3. Add in maple syrup and vanilla. Mix until dough is wet and sticks together.

4. Roll dough into small/medium sized balls, using hands. Option: roll dough balls in unsweetened coconut flakes, sesame seeds, or hemp hearts.

5. Place on baking sheet. Press down lightly with bottom of glass to create a flat top.

6. Bake for 10-12 minutes or until golden brown.

DECADENT CHOCOLATE AVOCADO MOUSSE
(Alexis)

Time:

1-2 hours and 20 minutes (20 minutes preparation, 1-2 hours setting)

Serves:

4-6

Ingredients:

6-8 chopped, pitted dates

3 avocados, pitted and scooped from skin

⅓ cup almond milk

2 tablespoons maple syrup

3 tablespoons cocoa powder

Directions:

1. Combine all ingredients in a blender until smooth.

2. Pour into small bowls or ramekins.

3. Place in fridge for 1-2 hours.

4. Top with whipped coconut cream and fruit and enjoy!

Recipes

PART 3

How does it work?

CHAPTER 5

The Hidden Organ: The Microbiome

The microbiome is a hot health topic in the news right now. It's been called the "hidden organ," because it remained unnoticed for many years. Technically, the microbiome is defined as all of the microorganisms that live in us or on us—including their genetic material. The vast majority of these microorganisms are the 30 trillion friendly bacteria that live in your lower gut. Many of these bacteria don't use oxygen, which has made them hard to culture and research, but the introduction of gene-sequencing gives scientists a new and relatively inexpensive tool with which to identify and study them. As a result, the microbiome is a very active area of medical research and the subject of hundreds of clinical trials.

We used to believe that all bacteria were harmful. And while it's true that certain virulent bacteria and viruses are capable of killing millions of people, it turns out that most of the 500 to 1000 species living in your gut are wonderfully beneficial.

What are the functions of your gut bacteria?

First, they help us to digest certain types of food. Most nutrients are digested and absorbed in your small intestine, but some foods cannot be digested by the enzymes present in the small intestine. Fruits and vegetables, for example, contain fiber that passes right through the small intestine, and goes into the large intestine, where your friendly bacteria digest them, and produce nutrients for cells in the lining of the gut.

A second function of your friendly gut bacteria is that they make important B vitamins—thiamine, riboflavin, nicotinic acid, pantothenic acid, pyridoxine, biotin, folate, and cobalamin or B_{12}. They also synthesize a certain type of vitamin K, which is vital for blood clotting factors, and they help the absorption of essential minerals like calcium, magnesium, and iron.

Their third important function is to helping to protect us from the invasion of harmful microorganisms. It turns out that 70-80% of your total immune system is located in the lining of the gut. Friendly bacteria occupy critical locations along your gut lining so that bad bacteria are prevented from crossing the gut barrier. The good guys also protect us by secreting antimicrobial chemicals to attack and destroy bad bacteria.

The fourth function is that they play a key role in the development of your gut lining. Without these friendly bacteria, certain gut immune and nerve cells do not mature properly, which jeopardizes the health of the entire gut lining.

The fifth (and wildest) function of your gut bacteria is that they produce critical substances that can cross the gut barrier and communicate with your brain and body, influencing digestion, appetite, state of mind—even turning genes on and off throughout your body. These bacteria are part of the *gut-brain axis*, which we will talk about later.

What factors can disrupt or change your gut bacteria?

The most important are:

- Caesarean birth

- Antibiotics

- Poor diet

- Medication

- Toxins

- Inadequate hygiene

- Lifestyle

- Age

Caesarean birth: The first bacteria that colonize the infant's gut are from the mother's skin and the hospital environment, and they are frequently not friendly bacteria. Studies show that children from caesarean births have a higher incidence of asthma, allergies, autoimmune diseases, and obesity in adulthood. In some countries, like China, over 50% of all births are caesarean. In private hospitals in Brazil, the number reaches 80%. Italy has the second highest caesarean birth rate in Europe with 38%, and over 30% of all births in the US are caesarean.

Antibiotics: A single dose can wipe out trillions of your helpful friendly bacteria. Most medical experts now agree that these wonder drugs have been massively overprescribed. One bad side effect of this is that certain bacteria have become resistant to antibiotics, posing a very real health threat, especially in hospitals.

How long does it take a damaged microbiome to recover from an antibiotic? Each person reacts differently. Some people can recover completely in a short time while others lose certain species of bacteria forever. Most doctors now recommend that we take probiotics after a course of antibiotics. But probiotics contain relatively few bacteria, so it is hard to understand how a few friendly bacteria are able to restore the enormous diversity of the hundreds of types of bacteria in your gut. Recent studies indicate that probiotics may not work in everyone and might even inhibit the growth of certain good bacteria.

Diet: Perhaps the most important factor which is able to change your gut bacteria is your diet. One excellent study examined gut bacteria in healthy children between ages one and six, living either in Europe (Italy) or in rural Africa (Burkina Faso), and found striking differences between the two ethnic and cultural groups. Scientists concluded that the most important factor causing these differences was the fiber content in the diet, which was almost twice as high in the children from Burkina Faso compared to the Italian children.

A number of studies have extended this research and consistently show that diet is the most critical factor in changing your microbial community. If you eat a vegetarian diet, certain kinds of bacteria will thrive. If you switch to meat, in a matter of days different varieties of bacteria will prosper.

Diet isn't the only thing that can alter the composition of your gut bacteria. Other factors, such as medication, infection, environmental toxins, whether we smoke or not, how much we exercise, your age, and even seasonal rhythms, can all affect your microbiome.

Hundreds of clinical studies are trying to find out whether a specific diet, probiotic, or lifestyle can help to cure specific diseases. There is even a new name, psychobiotics, for a type of probiotics that could treat mental and emotional disorders.

An entirely new field of medicine is emerging, which focuses exclusively on creating better health through the repair of your microbiome. One of the most important goals of the Rest and Repair Diet is to help reboot and restore this microbiome.

CHAPTER 6

Ayurveda and the Microbiome

With the discovery of the microbiome and the remarkable role your gut bacteria play in health and disease, it has recently become possible to better understand Ayurveda, the ancient health tradition of India, which has been practiced for many thousands of years. The Rest and Repair Diet includes many practical and effective recommendations from Ayurveda to help improve the state of your gut and microbiome.

Dosha and Prakriti

Ayurveda describes the mind and body in terms of three main underlying psychophysiological characteristics, or *doshas*, as they are traditionally referred to in Ayurveda. We use the term nature rather than dosha, because according to Ayurveda, you are born with a unique combination of Vata, Pitta, and Kapha, which is called your "Prakriti" or nature. (The state of your health at any one time is referred to as your "Vikriti.") By knowing both your Prakriti and Vikriti, an Ayurvedic physician can personalize your diet, lifestyle, and herbal supplements to prevent disease and create your best possible state of health.

Vata refers to systems of the body that control movement, such as your nervous system. Pitta refers to systems of the body concerned with metabolism, such as your digestive system. Kapha refers to systems involved with structure and lubrication, such as your bones and joints.

People with a Vata Prakriti or nature, have a variable digestion. When the Vata digestion is out of balance, they often become constipated, and may produce gas. Vata individuals tend to have a sensitive gut and are more susceptible to minor disruptions. Stress easily affects their mental state, causing worry, anxiety, and even fear.

Pittas have a strong digestion. If they are imbalanced or stressed, however, they can have a hyper-acidic stomach. In terms of emotional balance, the seemingly simple act of not eating on time can make them irritable, resulting in a condition that has come be known as "hangry."

Kaphas are described in Ayurveda as having a slower digestion and metabolism. When imbalanced, they can overeat and easily gain weight. An imbalance in Kapha can also lead to a lethargic and depressed state of mind.

Researchers who have studied predominantly Vata, Pitta, and Kapha individuals have found specific physiological and genetic differences. A recent study published in *Frontiers in Microbiology* showed that predominantly Vata, Pitta, or Kapha people also show a different composition of bacteria in their microbiome.

This finding is a huge breakthrough in the scientific understanding of Ayurveda.

Diet and Lifestyle

Ayurveda has always considered food as medicine and prescribes a specific diet and lifestyle for each individual. Ayurveda also uses spices and herbs to help create and maintain balance in the physiology, and to treat specific disorders.

Modern research has discovered many beneficial medicinal properties in Ayurvedic herbs and spices. Turmeric is one of the most well-studied medicinal plants in the Ayurvedic tradition. It has been the subject of thousands of peer-reviewed and published biomedical studies, with hundreds of potential preventive and therapeutic applications, as well as distinct beneficial physiological effects on such diseases as ulcerative colitis, stomach ulcers, osteoarthritis, heart disease, cancer, and neurodegenerative disorders. A number of studies also describe how turmeric interacts with the gut bacteria to modulate different aspects of the process of digestion.

Recent research shows that both ginger and an herbal preparation called triphala (composed of three different fruits) have a beneficial effect on your microbiome, increasing the number of friendly bacteria and decreasing the harmful ones.

Agni

In Ayurveda, *agni* means the fire of digestion, which can be understood in terms of the digestive enzymes that break down different foods, as well as enzymes controlling metabolism in different cells. The agni in your lower gut correlates with the gut bacteria present in the large intestine.

Ama

Ayurveda explains that most diseases are caused by an accumulation of *ama* or undigested food. This is similar to recent findings about "Leaky Gut Syndrome." In a leaky gut, the tight junctions that hold the cells of the gut wall together become loose, and as a result, undigested food and harmful substances "leak" through the gut wall and into the bloodstream, causing inflammation. Celiac disease is one of several conditions involving a leaky gut. We will go into the detail about Leaky Gut Syndrome in a later chapter.

If your agni is weak, ama accumulates and clogs your system, causing health problems. It is particularly harmful when it leaves the digestive system and enters other parts of the body, accumulating in the tissues. Symptoms of excess ama include fatigue and a feeling of heaviness, congestion, constipation, and mental confusion or "brain fog." Ayurveda considers excess ama to be the root cause of all disease.

Biorhythms

Ayurveda clearly identifies daily, seasonal, and lifetime rhythms. Each day, for example, consists of a sequence of periods, which are characterized by either Vata, Pitta, or Kapha. Each season is represented by either one dosha or a combination of doshas: Fall and winter are cold and dry, and correspond to the combination of Vata and Kapha dosha. Summer is hot and naturally corresponds to Pitta dosha. Spring is cold and wet, and corresponds to Kapha dosha.

Modern medicine recognizes the importance of daily rhythms to your health to such an extent that the 2017 Nobel Prize in Physiology and Medicine was awarded for research on the genetic basis of biological rhythms. From bacteria to humans, almost all forms of life have an internal "biological clock," which maintains an approximately 24-hour rhythm. When external signals of light and dark are introduced unnaturally, your master clock becomes confused and this creates health problems. Shift workers, for instance, have been shown to have a higher incidence of cancer, cardiovascular disease, digestive disorders, and obesity, as well as psychiatric and neurodegenerative diseases.

One of the most important timing issues for the body is *when* you eat. If you eat within 2 hours before you normally go to sleep, it can desynchronize the circadian rhythms of certain cells in the intestine and liver from those in the rest of your body.

Your gut bacteria also have biological rhythms. One scientific study created jet lag in mice by forcing these normally nocturnal animals to stay awake during the day. When the researchers transferred the gut bacteria from jet-lagged mice into germ-free mice, the recipient mice developed both obesity and glucose intolerance. Recent research on the gut bacteria reveals not only the presence of a daily rhythm, but also seasonal biorhythms—which again correlates with the ancient knowledge of Ayurveda.

Spring Detox

The Rest and Repair Diet is similar to a classic Ayurvedic Spring Detox Diet. Over the winter, Kapha and ama build up in your body. Spring is a period of awakening and renewal, and it is the ideal time to re-balance Kapha and reduce ama to prevent toxins and excess mucus from creating congestion and allergies. It is also the perfect time to reboot and increase your digestive fire or agni, detox your body, repair your gut, and eliminate any excess weight.

Foods that are primarily Kapha in nature—heavy, greasy, and mucus forming—tend to increase both Kapha and ama. During the Rest and Repair Diet it is important to reduce or eliminate such Kapha foods as milk products, wheat products, sugar, and red meat. If you would like to do a stricter Ayurvedic version of the diet, you can eliminate other heavy foods such as nut butters, eggs, chicken, and fish.

Kitchari, as we have mentioned, comes from Ayurveda and is one of the healthiest and most beneficial foods in the Rest and Repair Diet. It helps to detoxify and heal the gut. Leafy green vegetables are included because they are good detoxifiers, while heavier root vegetables should be eaten sparingly. It is helpful to note that the bitter, pungent, and astringent tastes of certain foods, spices, and herbs act as a powerful detoxing and cleansing combination. A bitter taste can dry and drain ama, while a pungent taste destroys and digests it. We will discuss the six Ayurveda tastes of Ayurveda in Chapter 8.

Probiotic Enemas and Bastis

Dr. David Perlmutter, a qualified neurologist with several best-selling books and a PBS series, talks about using probiotic enemas to help cure certain neurological disorders in his book *The Brain Maker.* Why should the average person tolerate the discomfort of an enema when probiotics can be taken orally? Probiotics that are taken orally must pass through your stomach and the small intestine, which is not ideal because stomach acid and digestive enzymes destroy many of the valuable probiotic bacteria long before they reach the colon. A probiotic enema, however, provides an almost instantaneous route to the colon, where most of your gut bacteria live.

Dr. Perlmutter describes Christopher, a teenage boy who had Tourette's syndrome since he was six. Tourette's patients typically have periodic spontaneous and uncontrollable movements, and they tend to repeat certain words or sounds. Over 100,000 children in the US have Tourette's, more than five times as many boys as girls. Although Christopher was able to attend school, by the time he was 13 he was suffering from the social stigma associated with his involuntary movements.

When Dr. Perlmutter interviewed Christopher's mother, facts came to light that pointed to his gut as the source of his disease. First, the boy's Tourette's symptoms worsened after eating specific foods, and secondly, Christopher had received numerous antibiotics when he was young.

Dr. Perlmutter reasoned that Christopher's medical history indicated a massive disruption of his gut bacteria and recommended that the boy take probiotic enemas rather than oral probiotics. The morning after Christopher's first probiotic enema, his mother called to report that her son's body had become noticeably calmer. Under Dr. Perlmutter's supervision, the treatment was continued daily and the probiotic dosage was increased to 1200 billion units. Christopher's Tourette's symptoms virtually disappeared. (Please note: It is important to have your doctor's approval before beginning a probiotic enema program.)

Many traditional systems of medicine, including Ayurveda, commonly use enemas. The Ayurvedic term for enema is *basti*, and bastis are a valuable part of the deep purification and detox treatment program known as *panchakarma*, which both cleanses the body of impurities and promotes health and longevity.

There are many different types of bastis: some are for purification, others for elimination, still others strengthen the tissues and provide valuable nutrients. Bastis use ingredients like sesame oil, medicated ghee, buttermilk, lassi, many different combinations of herbs, and in special cases, bone broth. The ancient Ayurvedic doctors understood the importance of the digestive system and how to quickly rebalance and help repair it by introducing herbs and oils directly into the colon.

Ojas

According to Ayurveda, the digestion and gut play leading roles in your immunity. Ayurveda speaks about a substance called Ojas, *the finest product of digestion*, which strengthens the immune system and has many beneficial effects on the mind and body.

How can Ojas be identified in terms of modern science? There are many possible candidates for this extraordinary substance. One possibility is serotonin, a key regulator of mood, sleep, appetite, and other brain functions. Your gut produces 90% of all your serotonin, which circulates throughout your bloodstream and influences not only your immune system, but your heart rate, blood clotting, intestinal motility, pulmonary arteries, heart, brain, and mammary glands, as well as the cell growth of liver and bone cells. Another interesting candidate is a chemical called butyric acid, which is produced by the gut bacteria and has numerous beneficial effects, including the improvement of immunity. There are many other possible choices for Ojas, but we will have to wait for conclusive research to finally discover this unique Ayurvedic substance.

Maharishi AyurVeda

Maharishi Mahesh Yogi is the founder of the Transcendental Meditation program. He also spent many years revitalizing Ayurveda, and reintroducing specific techniques for the development of consciousness. It is in his honor that a new body of knowledge referred to as Maharishi AyurVeda was named.

Meditation is an integral part of Ayurveda and its sister discipline, Yoga. The practice of the Transcendental Meditation (TM) program, introduced by Maharishi over fifty years ago, has been shown to have beneficial effects on mental and physical health. Over $25 million in grants from the National Institutes of Health have supported research that demonstrates the positive effects of TM on cardiovascular disease. One of the most prominent studies reports a 48% reduction in heart attacks, strokes, and deaths in the TM group, as compared to randomly assigned controls.

Maharishi was also responsible for the revival of the ancient practice of pulse diagnosis, which is a highly sophisticated diagnostic tool of Ayurveda. Even a beginning practitioner of Ayurveda, however, can learn the practice of simple self-pulse diagnosis, which is an excellent way to immediately become aware of imbalances in your physiology before they manifest into disease.

The knowledge of Maharishi AyurVeda can be learned through continuing education online courses and degree programs at Maharishi University of Management (MUM), an accredited university located in Fairfield, Iowa.

Gut/Brain Nature

We use the term Gut/Brain Nature, rather than dosha or prakriti, in order to emphasize the importance of the gut-brain axis to your health. We suggest that you take a simple online quiz (at doc-gut.com), based on the principles of Ayurveda, to help determine your own Gut/Brain Nature. (See Chapter 21 for specific diets for your Gut/Brain Nature.)

CHAPTER 7

The Diet War

America is in the middle of a huge diet war. Should we follow a Mediterranean, Paleo, Vegan, or a Ketogenic diet? The *US News and World Report* do not give a high rating to more radical diets like the Paleo or Keto diet, and consider the DASH and Mediterranean diets as the healthiest.

DASH stands for Dietary Approach to Stop Hypertension, and includes lots of fruits, vegetables, whole grains, lean proteins, and low-fat dairy. It also recommends reducing salt, saturated fats, and high-sugar or artificially sweetened drinks. The Mediterranean diet is similar, with a few variations. The main feature of the Mediterranean diet consists of olive oil, legumes, unrefined cereals, fruits, and vegetables, with a moderate consumption of fish, dairy products (mostly as cheese and yogurt), wine, and fewer meat products.

Alternative health experts disagree with the *US News and World Report's* ratings. Dr. David Perlmutter, who we mentioned earlier, warns about the perils of modern wheat and recommends a completely gluten-free diet. He also explains why cholesterol is critical for your brain, citing many studies that disagree with the long-cherished belief that fat and cholesterol are bad for your health.

Dr. Josh Axe is a popular alternative health expert who promotes a Paleo-type diet, which eliminate foods that he feels damage your gut health, such as wheat, commercial cow's milk, sugar, hydrogenated oils, foods that have been genetically modified (GM), and processed food and beverages.

Dr. Joseph Mercola is a long-established alternative health expert who has written a number of best-selling books. In his latest, *Fat for Fuel*, he promotes a Keto diet and shows how the food industry has influenced scientific research on food and US dietary recommendations for many decades. As a result, Americans have been eating food that isn't good for us, like trans fats and sugar, and avoiding foods with healthy fats, which are critical to your mental and physical health.

The recommendations of these alternative health experts have several features in common, including the elimination of the following foods:

- Gluten

- Dairy

- Sugar

Sound familiar? It should, because this is an important part of the Rest and Repair Diet. The main difference between the Rest and Repair Diet and some of the more radical diets proposed by alternative health experts is the *duration* of the diet. The Rest and Repair Diet eliminates gluten, dairy, and sugar for only 3 weeks. When you reintroduce them in the Self Discovery program, you can then decide if you want to continue to keep them out of your diet.

CHAPTER 8

Appetite and Cravings

Is your gut bacteria craving chocolate ice cream, or is it your brain?

Your appetite is regulated by centers in your brain, but there are also many different chemicals in the bloodstream that influence the brain. The most important of these are two hormones, ghrelin and leptin. Ghrelin is known as the "hunger hormone," while leptin is the "satiety hormone." Ghrelin is your "ON" switch for eating. It activates centers in your brain that *stimulate appetite.* Leptin is the "OFF" switch, which stimulates brain centers that *decrease appetite.*

If you haven't eaten anything for a while before you started reading this, then ghrelin is being produced in your stomach and will eventually tell your brain: "Eat Now." If you had something to eat recently and you are feeling full, then leptin is being produced by your fat cells, and it's telling your brain: "No snacks. Thanks anyway."

The modern world creates complications for these hormones. If you stay up late, for example, and don't get enough sleep, leptin will *decrease* and you will tend to eat more. Of course, you will eventually gain weight. This is just one example. There are many things you do that can mess up the inner intelligence of your body.

What is the role of your gut bacteria in weight gain or loss? It turns out that your gut bacteria produce hormones and chemicals that are very similar to leptin and ghrelin. Gut bacteria can communicate or "talk" to your brain, by means of a variety of chemicals and nerve fibers. Why do they do this? Because the food you eat helps to determine which species of bacteria thrive and dominate in your gut. Your gut bacteria, therefore, have a strong evolutionary motivation to influence your food choices. A number of research papers even suggest that they determine what you eat!

What does Ayurveda say about appetite? Ayurveda recommends listening to your body and eating only when you are hungry. Ayurveda, as you know, also places almost as much emphasis on *how* you eat as *what* you eat.

Ayurveda recommends having the following six tastes at each meal: sweet, salty, sour, bitter, pungent, and astringent. You will be surprised to learn that the *sweet* taste can be satisfied with foods other than sugar, such as rice, dates, even licorice root. *Salty* foods include different types of salt, black olives, and tamari. Some examples of *sour* are lemons, vinegar, and pickled or fermented foods. *Bitter* taste includes green vegetables, turmeric, and many green and black teas. Examples of *pungent* foods are hot spices, ginger, and onions. Finally, some *astringent* foods are pomegranates, cranberries, and okra. Ayurveda tells us that some of your cravings occur because not all of the six tastes were present in your meals.

How does modern science explain cravings? Cravings are considered to be "learned behaviors," which often involve the desire for a specific food, activity, or drug. Are cravings considered addictive? Not everyone agrees, but many suggest that cravings are strong memories linked to a certain psychological need. One book that explains cravings is *The Prime* by Dr. Kulreet Chaudhary, a highly qualified neurologist, trained in Ayurveda and Integrative Medicine. She uses the example of the craving for addictive drugs. Certain drugs can cause the release of the neurotransmitter dopamine in reward centers in the brain, causing a feeling of pleasure. If more drugs are taken, the brain adapts by reducing the number of dopamine receptors to protect itself from being overwhelmed. The unfortunate end result is that even more drugs are needed to produce the same effect and the person gradually becomes addicted, experiencing terrible withdrawal symptoms if they stop taking the drug.

Dr. Chaudhary suggests that similar processes take place when you crave sugar. Your brain experiences pleasure and physically adapts, so that you must eat more and more sugar in order to have the same effect. You then start to gain weight, and may reach an obese state, resulting in health problems, such as diabetes or cardiovascular disease. Dr. Chaudhary explains that if you detoxify your body and change your diet for a long enough period, your brain will adapt and return to a normal healthy balanced state, and cravings will reduce significantly. She recommends systematically detoxing the body with Ayurvedic Digest and Detox Tea and using herbs such as Ashwagandha and Brahmi to help subdue cravings.

What is the role of your gut bacteria in cravings and addiction? Recent research suggests that gut bacteria can influence the brain pathways involved in eating disorders and in alcohol and drug addiction. Animal and human studies have uncovered potential mechanisms by which the gut bacteria influence all of these problems. Research is now underway to determine how positive changes in your gut bacteria can help to reduce cravings and addictions.

The next time you reach for a chocolate truffle ice cream cone with sprinkles—blame it on your gut bacteria.

CHAPTER 9

Digestion

A history tale is often told to medical students studying the digestive system. In 1911, two competing groups, the Norwegians and British, attempted to be first to reach the geographic South Pole. Explorer Roald Amundsen led the Norwegian team. Amundsen prepared by studying strategies used by the Inuits in their hunting trips. For example, he used sleds, skis, and dogs to travel on land, and supplemented his supplies with fresh meat. The Norwegian team reached the South Pole first and everyone returned safely.

The British, lead by Captain Robert Scott, attempted a more modern scientific approach using specially prepared foods, consisting of carbohydrates, proteins, and fats. Their transportation included motor sledges, the height of technology at the time, along with ponies and dogs. The British team also reached the South Pole, but none of them returned. Each of the five members died at different times and from different complications. They had adequate rations for a good part of the journey, but their food lacked key vitamins, which over time caused severe health problems and ultimately death. The lesson the medical students had to learn from this story is the critical importance of vitamins.

Digestion involves the breaking down of foods into their simplest components, and then the absorption of vital nutrients, such as vitamins, into our bloodstream. Many parts of your body are involved in digestion: centers in the brain, organs of the digestive system, digestive enzymes secreted by the pancreas, bile made by the liver, and, of course, the gut bacteria in your large intestine.

A typical American meal might consist of meat, potatoes, a few vegetables, and possibly a salad. The potatoes and vegetables are mostly made of carbohydrates formed by long chains of sugar molecules. In order for carbohydrates to be absorbed in the body, they need to be broken down into simple sugars.

Meat is mainly protein, which consists of chains of amino acids held together by special chemical bonds. Proteins need to be broken down into simple amino acids before they can be absorbed by the cells of your small intestine.

This meal will also have some fats from the meat or from butter added to the potatoes. Fats have to first be emulsified and then broken down into simple fatty acids before they can be absorbed by the cells in your small intestine.

Minerals and vitamins are absorbed by the cells of your gut, but in some cases, special factors are involved. As we learned from the story of the South Pole, it isn't enough to eat carbohydrates, fats, proteins, and minerals—you need vitamins to be healthy.

Your mouth secretes an enzyme called amylase, which helps to digest carbohydrates as they travel through the esophagus and into your stomach. Your stomach is important for the digestion of proteins, and allows for the temporary storage of food before it descends into your small intestine. In the small intestine, various enzymes are produced that allow proteins, fats, and carbohydrates to be digested. Other enzymes are made in your pancreas and then secreted into the small intestine. The process of breaking down fat is aided by bile salts that are made in your liver and stored in the gall bladder.

The walls of your small intestine are formed in a series of "bumps," called villi. Each of these bumps consists of a continuous series of cells lining the small intestine. Most of the cells are special absorptive cells, but some have other functions, such as the secretion of mucus and bacteria-killing substances to protect the lining of the gut.

There are even smaller bumps called microvilli on the special absorptive cells in the small intestine. The purpose of this unique landscape of "bumps within bumps" is to provide the largest possible surface area for the absorption of nutrients. If you were to spread out the lining of your small intestine, it would be about the size of half a tennis court.

How does your body selectively bring in nutrients that are good for you and keep out harmful bacteria? The cells in your intestinal wall are tightly linked together so that bacteria cannot enter the bloodstream. There are specific channels or gates on the surface of special absorptive cells that only allow certain nutrients into the cells. The nutrients then pass from inside the cell and into the bloodstream, which carries them to the liver and other areas to be metabolized and processed. Fats are unique because they move directly from special absorptive cells into the lymph system, and then enter the bloodstream.

Only the lettuce in the salad of the typical American meal cannot be digested in the small intestine. Lettuce contains fiber, a type of carbohydrate, but our body does not produce the right enzymes to break it down. Instead, it passes to the large intestine, where it is digested by your bacteria. The large intestine absorbs any excess water or minerals and it is the place where waste materials are stored before being eliminated.

One purpose of the Rest and Repair Diet is to improve your digestion by repairing your gut lining and rebooting the microbiome.

CHAPTER 10

Leaky Gut

The term Leaky Gut Syndrome covers a range of digestive symptoms that include gas, bloating, cramps, nausea, indigestion, heartburn, and food sensitivity. Much of what is now understood about a leaky gut comes from the work of Dr. Alessio Fasano, one of the world's leading experts on celiac disease.

Dr. Fasano has shown that gluten in wheat contains a short protein called gliadin, which triggers a series of biochemical events that cause a leaky gut. The cells that line the walls of the small intestine are normally held together by tight junctions (which consist of specialized proteins that bind the cells as a rope might bind two pieces of wood). In a healthy state, the tight junctions allow only water and small particles to go from the gut into your bloodstream and throughout your body. But when you eat wheat, the gliadin causes these junctions to momentarily come apart.

In celiac patients, even a tiny amount of gluten and gliadin can trigger a long-term opening in the tight junctions, which creates a "leaky gut." When the gut lining is breached, larger molecules and even bacteria can enter your bloodstream and cause an inflammatory response. If a celiac patient continues to consume foods that contain gluten, the result will be chronic inflammation and even a full-blown autoimmune response, during which the immune system becomes so agitated that it begins to attack normal healthy tissues in the body. The only real solution for a celiac patient is to stop eating anything containing gluten (wheat, barley, rye, etc.).

In Ayurveda, as we have mentioned, there is a concept similar to leaky gut. If the agni is weak and food is not properly digested, you produce ama or undigested food, which can leak into your bloodstream. The accumulation of ama in different tissues is considered to be the cause of many diseases.

Your gut lining is constantly under attack from harmful bacteria inside the gut. Beneath the cells that line the gut there are blood vessels, nerves, and most importantly, immune cells—the warriors of your gut, who attack any bacteria that might sneak through a tight junction or into a cell membrane.

The gut contains 70-80% of all the cells in your immune system. There are even small "forts" along the gut barrier, called Peyer's patches, that are loaded with immune cells. Also present are M cells (microfold cells), which act as "scouts" that identify and "interrogate" harmful bacteria. Once bad bacteria are identified, they are marked for destruction and eliminated in a massive battle, which employs lethal chemicals secreted by your gut immune cells.

What happens when bacteria get through your gut wall? Everyone knows how easy it is to come down with a sudden attack of diarrhea, especially in some foreign countries. These uncomfortable conditions are caused when a bacteria is able to trick the body's defenses and, at least temporarily, overwhelm the gut barrier defense system. Cholera is one of the most severe examples. Caused by the bacteria *Vibrio cholera,* it results in a huge loss of bodily fluids. The *Vibrio cholera* bacteria penetrates the acid environment of the stomach and lodges itself in the walls of the small intestine, where it produces a toxin that causes the tight junctions to open up, and a massive amount of water moves from inside the body into the gut, resulting in severe diarrhea.

A great deal of research is now focused on the gut barrier and the role your friendly gut bacteria play in maintaining its integrity. Many experts recommend probiotics and specific diets to enhance the defenses of the gut barrier. The primary focus of the Rest and Repair Diet is to repair a leaky gut and help your microbiome reboot itself so that friendly bacteria can better help defend your body.

CHAPTER 11

Stress and the Gut-Brain Axis

Stress affects everyone. Each psychological state you experience in life has a corresponding physiological state. One of the ways stress affects people is through a complex network called the gut-brain axis, which has an enormous impact on the health of your body and mind. The gut-brain axis consists of a number of major systems: the nervous system, enteric nervous system or ENS, endocrine system, immune system, and the gut bacteria.

Most people know about the fight or flight response, and for many of you, this response is turned on needlessly and too frequently, with the result that your body and mind are in a constant state of over-excitation. This hyper state of your nervous system is linked to a number of diseases; digestive disorders are near the top of the list.

During stressful situations, your brain has various ways of disrupting your gut. It can send signals directly through nerves or through hormones and chemical messengers. During stress, for example, the brain triggers your adrenal glands to release the stress hormone cortisol, which goes into your bloodstream and affects both the gut itself and the gut bacteria. Cortisol can increase intestinal permeability, which results in a leaky gut. It can also shut down the activity of the gut immune system.

The part of the gut-brain axis most people are unfamiliar with is the enteric nervous system (ENS), which acts as a "second nervous system" inside your gut. Your ENS monitors and regulates your gut, sending signals to your brain about every detail of digestion. The ENS produces more than 30 neurotransmitters, and many are the same as those in the brain. Almost 90% of all the serotonin in your body is produced by cells in the gut, as well as 50% of the dopamine. Stress disrupts the important activities of your ENS, and contributes to various digestive problems.

There is a two-way communication between the gut and the brain. Stress in your brain can disrupt your digestive process, while stress in your gut can disrupt your mind and emotions.

Gut bacteria use the vagus nerve to communicate with your brain, and also to produce a wide variety of chemical messengers, including neurotransmitters and hormones that can enter the bloodstream and affect parts of your brain. Brain imaging has shown that people react differently to stress, *depending on the type of bacteria in their gut*. Subjects receiving a probiotic showed a reduced stress response, with less activity in the emotional areas of the brain.

What can we do to counter the damaging effects of stress? Traditional systems of medicine, including Ayurveda, contain a wealth of time-tested procedures to reduce stress and improve the state of your gut. The Transcendental Meditation (TM) program, for example, has a remarkable ability to reduce the effects of stress, and to decrease the incidence of stress-related disease, including digestive disorders.

Ayurveda, which incorporates meditation and yoga, also uses specific diets and herbs to reduce the effects of stress on the gut. We have mentioned that the Rest and Repair Diet is similar to an Ayurvedic Spring detox diet and also how different Ayurvedic herbs help to strengthen good bacteria and eliminate harmful bacteria. Once you realize how important the gut-brain axis is to your mental and physical health, you can understand the value of repairing your gut and rebooting your microbiome.

CHAPTER 12

Mental Health and Neurological Disorders

Research shows that gut bacteria affect two of the most prevalent mental disorders, anxiety and depression. According to the World Health Organization, between 1990 and 2013, the number of people suffering from incapacitating depression and/or anxiety rose from 416 million to 615 million. The most common treatment for anxiety and depression is prescription medication, which often has side-effects. Wouldn't you prefer a truly natural remedy if it had the same or better result?

In 2011, a group of scientists in Ireland and Canada developed an interesting model for studying the effects of gut bacteria on the mental health of mice. The animals were subjected to a stress test, during which they were forced to swim in an environment with no escape (not something mice or any other beings enjoy doing). The scientists then measured what they called "behavioral despair." This same test was used to assess antidepressant drugs.

The scientists found that mice fed a probiotic broth for several weeks before the test were able to swim longer and showed less behavioral despair. This led the researchers to hypothesize that the bacteria of the mice were somehow altering the chemical environment of their brain, the way a drug might. Studies show that patients with depression have different types of gut bacteria from normal patients.

In her book, *Gut and Psychology Syndrome*, Dr. Natasha Campbell-McBride states that in her clinical experience, she has yet to meet a child with autism, hyperactivity, the inability to learn, or mood and behavioral disorders, *who does not have some gut abnormalities*. The digestive system, she says, is the key to a child's mental development. Other doctors and scientists have also made this important observation.

In 2013, it was estimated that Autism Spectrum Disorder, or ASD, affects over 20 million people, and the number keeps growing. The evidence that ASD is caused or influenced by diet or abnormal gut bacteria is still controversial. Most scientists believe that ASD is the result of genetic and environmental influences. Many animal studies, however, strongly implicate gut bacteria as an important factor.

In one study, a group of female mice were given a high-fat diet in order to induce autistic behavior in their offspring, while another group ate normally. When the over-fed mothers bred and bore offspring, their babies showed behavioral traits similar to autism, spending less time with other mice and displaying abnormal social interactions. Investigators then looked at the composition of the gut bacteria in the two groups and clear differences were found. When the autistic-like mice consumed a probiotic, important aspects of their social behavior became normal.

One of the most interesting speculations on how the gut bacteria may affect mental disease is in an article called *Bread and Other Edible Agents of Mental Disease*, by two professors from Padua, Italy. They talk about morphine-like substances called exorphins, which are produced from gluten and milk when they are improperly digested. These substances can be both addictive and hallucinogenic.

You may have heard something about endorphins, which are the body's natural painkillers, said to be responsible for a "runner's high." Exorphins are similar to endorphins in that they fit into an opioid receptor, but they are different because they are not naturally produced in the body and come from an external source (like gluten or milk). The Italian researchers suggest that exorphins might be the cause of certain mental conditions, including schizophrenia. They cite case studies of schizophrenic patients who became markedly better when they went on a diet that excluded gluten and milk. It is very interesting and perhaps indicative of human nature, however, that patients refused to continue this Spartan diet even though it made them feel better.

The Rest and Repair Diet is not meant to cure specific mental or other disorders. Subjectively, however, many people report improvements in clarity of mind.

CHAPTER 13

Intestinal Disorders

Irritable Bowel Syndrome

Between 25 and 45 million people in the US have irritable bowel syndrome or IBS. Symptoms include abdominal pain, bloating, gas, diarrhea, and constipation. Stress is a critical factor that can trigger symptoms and make the condition worse. IBS affects people of all ages, but 2 out of 3 patients are women.

A recent analysis of IBS suggests that it may be caused and aggravated by a disruption in the gut bacteria. The good news is that studies show that probiotics can improve some of the symptoms of IBS.

Inflammatory Bowel Disease

Over one million people in this country suffer from inflammatory bowel disease or IBD. The two main types of IBD are ulcerative colitis (UC) and Crohn's disease. Both conditions cause severe inflammation in the gut lining, but UC damages only the colon and rectum, while Crohn's disease can injure any part of the digestive tract.

The exact cause of inflammatory bowel disease is unknown, although recent theories suggest a complex interaction between stress, genetics, and the disruption of gut bacteria. Symptoms worsen in the presence of antibiotics, infection, poor diet, drugs, smoking, and stress.

Research shows that probiotics can improve IBD, although the results are not as consistent as with IBS. One study reported improvements with a probiotic cocktail of about 17 strains of a particular type of bacteria.

In the case of Crohn's disease, doctors have had temporary success with a special diet called exclusive enteral nutrition or EEN—which involves a complete liquid diet using a special formula. This diet has been found to induce remission in Crohn's disease, especially in children and adolescents.

Celiac Disease

The University of Chicago Celiac Disease Center estimates that at least three million people in the US are living with celiac disease right now and 97% of them are undiagnosed. A related condition, called non-celiac gluten sensitivity, affects about 6% of the population.

Celiac disease has over 300 different symptoms, from mild to extreme. Some of the most frequently reported are: abdominal pain, nausea, anemia, an itchy blistery rash, loss of bone density, headaches, general fatigue, bone or joint pain, mouth ulcers, weight loss, and heartburn.

SIBO

SIBO stands for Small Intestinal Bacterial Overgrowth. Normally, there are only a few bacteria in the small intestine, but with this condition, there is an overgrowth of bacteria, which start fermenting food before it is digested or passed to the lower gut. The result is excess gas, bloating, and burping, and valuable nutrients may not be effectively absorbed.

To test for SIBO a standard hydrogen breath test can be taken at home or at a doctor's office. The problem is that this test is not perfect, detecting only about 60% of SIBO cases.

Up to now, the standard treatment for SIBO has been antibiotics, but many experts feel that *probiotics should be the first line of treatment*, followed by antibiotics only if necessary. One of the most interesting new treatments is the use of herbal preparations. *A carefully controlled study showed that several commercial herbal products were as effective as an antibiotic.*

Again the Rest and Repair Diet is not meant to cure specific intestinal disorders, but subjectively, people report improvements in digestion and gut comfort.

CHAPTER 14

Other Diseases

Chronic inflammation is rampant in the modern world and lies at the basis of many diseases, particularly autoimmune disease. New research suggests that chronic inflammation begins as a localized response in your gut, which activates certain immune cells. These immune cells then set off a chain reaction that leads to inflammation in other organs of the body. The long list of diseases believed to be caused by gut inflammation includes: diabetes, rheumatoid arthritis, high blood pressure, metabolic syndrome, respiratory disease, stroke, and cancer.

Let's briefly consider some of the most interesting research on these conditions. High blood pressure affects over 1 billion people around the world. In an extraordinary study at the Johns Hopkins University School of Medicine, the gut bacteria were shown to produce substances that influence the kidney to *help lower blood pressure*. Numerous other studies demonstrated that probiotics can marginally help patients with both high blood pressure and type 2 diabetes.

Research on 900 subjects in the Netherlands found that the gut bacteria are strongly linked to healthy levels of good cholesterol (HDL) and triglycerides. The scientists concluded that altering gut bacteria might be a new way to improve blood cholesterol levels. Metabolic syndrome is the combination of a number of cardiovascular risk factors, such as high blood pressure, abnormal cholesterol levels, diabetes, and obesity. Evidence strongly suggests that altering bacteria can improve metabolic syndrome.

Respiratory diseases have also been associated with gut problems. When the health records of almost 2 million children in Denmark were examined over a 35-year period, it was found that the risk of developing asthma after a caesarean birth is 20% higher than after a normal birth. Research on the effects of probiotics and prebiotics on asthma and allergies have shown some positive results, although conclusions are mixed.

Another interesting finding is that gut bacteria can influence the severity of a stroke, the second leading cause of death worldwide. Gut bacteria may even affect cancer. Animal studies show that certain beneficial bacteria can help to delay and slow down the onset of cancer in cells of the immune system. Gut bacteria have also been found to make one anti-cancer drug twice as effective at reducing tumors.

Probably the most surprising and widely accepted medical treatment that has arisen as a result of research on the microbiome is fecal transplant. This involves taking a feces sample from a healthy individual and transplanting it into an unhealthy person. The procedure is widely used in hospitals today for *Clostridium difficile* infection, a life threatening and often recurring condition. In some studies, this treatment has been shown to be 90% effective, which is far better than antibiotic treatment.

One of the most provocative experiments is on the effect of gut bacteria on obesity, which we know is a growing problem today and a major risk factor for both diabetes and heart disease. Fecal transplants were taken from a pair of human twins—one who was obese, the other lean. The two fecal transplants were given to two groups of mice. The mice that received the transplant from the obese human twin gained weight, while the mice receiving microbes from the lean sibling lost weight.

Most people agree that fecal transplant is an "unpleasant" approach to curing disease. However, these experiments have alerted medical experts to the possibility of using fecal transplants and oral probiotics to help cure chronic disease.

Diet has long been a topic of great interest in the study of chronic disease; however, there is still no clear conclusion about what the best diet is for specific diseases. If anything, the battle between conventional medicine and alternative health care is more heated than ever, especially over the role of fats in cardiovascular disease.

The Rest and Repair Diet is not meant to treat a specific disorder. It is designed to help repair the gut lining and restore the microbiome by combining the traditional knowledge of Ayurveda with the latest findings in modern and alternative health treatment.

CHAPTER 15

Sugar

Let's talk about sugar. Most of us like it, some of us love it. Health experts strongly believe that we eat too much. Some even think that it is the main cause of chronic inflammation.

If you Google the words "sugar" and "inflammation," two opposing views will appear on the first page. One article is: *Does Sugar Cause Inflammation in the Body?* by Mary Jane Brown, PhD, a registered dietitian. Containing 47 excellent scientific references, this article presents a convincing case that yes, sugar does cause inflammation.

A second article, which appears a little lower down on the list, is *Inflammatory Claims about Inflammation* by Jeff Schweitzer, PhD, a former Assistant Director for International Affairs in the Office of Science and Technology Policy in the Clinton administration. Dr. Schweitzer argues that health experts are making pseudoscientific assertions about inflammation. He acknowledges that if we eat too much sugar in one sitting, along with large amounts of saturated fats, the result could be an acute inflammatory response.

However, he strongly objects to claims linking sugar to chronic inflammation.

What can we conclude from these conflicting opinions? No one experiment tells the whole story. The ambiguities in the research findings have lead to different opinions on the effects of sugar on your health and you should be aware that these opinions have been influenced by the sugar industry.

In his book, *The Case Against Sugar*, Gary Taubes explains that for decades, the sugar lobby funded researchers to place the blame for increased cardiovascular disease on excess saturated fat, rather than on sugar. One of the most prominent researchers was Ancil Keys, who appeared on the cover of *Time* magazine in 1961 as the nation's leading expert on nutrition. When John Yudkin, a British physiologist and nutritionist, and the founding Professor of the Department of Nutrition at Queen Elizabeth College in London, tried to alert the world to the potential dangers of excess sugar, Keys and the sugar lobby managed to destroy Yudkin's credibility. Ancil Keys' studies on fat intake and heart disease had an enormous influence on US government nutritional guidelines. Now we know that Keys cherry-picked data to support his theories and left out important conflicting information.

A recent paper published by researchers from the University of California, San Francisco, has exposed how a trade group called the Sugar Research Foundation, known today as the Sugar Association, paid scientists in the 1960s to publish an influential review of research on sugar, fat, and heart disease. Two of these paid scientists were Dr. Mark Hegsted, who became head of the United

States Department of Agriculture, and Dr. Fredrick J. Stare, the chairman of Harvard's nutrition department. In this way, the sugar industry has indirectly had a major impact on the federal government's dietary guidelines, which called for a reduction in dietary fat intake, but no change in sugar intake.

There was more than one negative consequence to these recommendations. First, the food industry created trans fats, which were later discovered to be bad for your health. Second, the food industry started to add sugar and salt to virtually all processed foods to improve the taste. Third, in order to stabilize sugar prices, the food industry invented high fructose corn syrup, which many alternative health experts strongly agree to be detrimental to your health.

Robert Lustig, MD, Professor of Pediatrics in the Division of Endocrinology at the University of California, San Francisco, is one of the leading proponents against sugar, especially high fructose corn syrup. In the YouTube video *Sugar: The Bitter Truth*, seen by millions of viewers, he talks about why sugar is toxic to the body.

The American Heart Association eventually conducted a highly comprehensive study on sugar, which led to the conclusion that excess sugar increases the risk of developing obesity, cardiovascular disease, hypertension, and obesity–related cancers. They now recommend that children consume less sugar as part of a healthier diet.

Shamefully, the food industry still helps fund many important health associations, such as the American Heart Association and the American Diabetic Association. Last year, an article in

The New York Times revealed that Coca-Cola, the world's largest producer of sugary beverages, has provided millions of dollars in funding for researchers to play down the link between sugary drinks and obesity.

The Rest and Repair Diet asks you to cut back or eliminate sugar for a 3-week period, and then reintroduce it if you wish. Each person has a unique physiology and it is important for you to become aware of how sugar affects your mind and body.

CHAPTER 16

Dairy

Welcome to the Dairy Wars. If you look up the words "dairy" and "inflammation" on a search engine, you will again find contradictory research papers and blogs. Some experts are adamant that dairy causes inflammation. Others dismiss the idea as unscientific, citing recent review articles, which actually state that dairy is largely neutral and even anti-inflammatory.

The few natural components in dairy products most likely to cause inflammation are sugar (lactose), and protein (specifically casein and whey).

Dairy Sugar

Lactose is composed of two simple sugars, glucose and galactose. When you are a baby, you produce an enzyme called lactase, which breaks the lactose into glucose and galactose—a necessary step to allow these sugars to be absorbed into the cells of your small intestine. In time, however, and depending on their genetic make up, many people stop making the enzyme lactase.

About 65% of today's world population cannot digest lactose, a condition called lactose intolerance.

Why is lactose intolerance a problem?

If lactose isn't digested in the small intestine, it goes to the large intestine, where it is fermented by the gut bacteria. The result is excess gas, causing abdominal pain, bloating, and other intestinal problems.

How common is lactose intolerance in the US?

Approximately 75% of all African Americans, Native Americans, and Jewish Americans are lactose intolerant, along with 50% Mexican Americans and 90% of Asian Americans.

Who can digest milk?

About 90% of Americans of Northern European descent are able to produce the enzyme lactase even as adults, and are, therefore, able to absorb the milk sugar into their bloodstream.

How can a person cope with lactose intolerance?

These days it's easy to switch to lactose-free milk, or plant-based "milks," such as soy, nut, rice, and coconut milks. Butter, cheese, and yogurt can usually be tolerated in moderate amounts because the lactose has been removed from these products when they are made. Some experts suggest that probiotic foods like yogurt help alleviate symptoms of lactose intolerance by altering the composition of the gut bacteria in the lower intestine.

Dairy Proteins

The other elements in dairy products that may cause inflammation are the proteins casein and whey. And the most obvious type of inflammation caused by these proteins is a milk allergy, which is a serious inflammatory reaction. Symptoms of a milk allergy include: throat or tongue swelling, shortness of breath, vomiting, lightheadedness, low blood pressure, and even an itchy rash. Milk allergies are present in 1% to 3% of the world's population. If you think that you might have a milk allergy, it is important for you to be properly tested and diagnosed. Six major allergenic proteins have been identified in cow's milk as the cause of a milk allergy (four are from casein, and two from whey).

The amount of casein protein varies in different types of milk. In cow's milk, casein is nearly 80% of the protein. In human milk, it makes up only 40% of the protein. Casein is found in cheese and is also used as a food additive. There are two distinct types of casein—A1 and A2 beta-casein—and the difference between these two is an area of great controversy.

Scientists believe that this difference is the result of a genetic mutation in cows, which occurred when cattle were first brought into Europe 5,000 to 10,000 years ago. Modern day cows in Europe (with the exception of France), the United States, Australia, and New Zealand produce a mixture of A1 and A2 beta-casein. In Asia and Africa most cows produce only the A2 beta-casein. Breeds such as Jersey, Guernsey, Asian cows, and others (sheep, goats, etc.), produce mostly A2 beta-casein, while Holstein,

Friesian, Ayrshire, and British Shorthorn breeds produce equal amounts of A1 and A2 beta-casein. Human milk contains A2 beta-casein.

The difference between A1 and A2 milk was brought to public attention when a company in New Zealand, the *a2 Milk Company* (previously called A2 Corporation) made claims that A1 milk was responsible for a number of diseases. They have since been forced to withdraw these claims, and in 2009, the European Food Safety Authority (EFSA) reviewed the scientific literature and found no relationship between chronic diseases and A1 milk.

But the Dairy War is not over. Recent studies in China found that there are a number of benefits from A2 milk, compared to A1 milk, in terms of digestive discomfort and elimination. However, it should be noted that the researchers involved in these studies were supported by the a2 Milk Company. (The a2 Milk Company produces A2 milk!)

Another type of protein found in milk is from whey, which has become a popular protein supplement for athletes. Again, the potential benefits of whey are not without debate.

There are other issues with milk, including contamination by hormones, antibiotics, and other substances, as well as the question of how pasteurization and homogenization affect the quality of milk.

Dairy products have been an integral part of many great traditions of health, including Ayurveda, yet a large part of the population of India is lactose intolerant. The resolution of this seeming paradox may lie in the way dairy products are prepared and consumed. For example, until recently, most dairy products in India were fermented to make either yogurt (and lassi) or *panir* (a type of cheese). Historically, much of India has followed the Ayurvedic recommendation that milk should always be boiled, and that certain digestive spices, such as ginger and cardamom, be added.

As we often point out, each individual is different and there may be periods in your life during which you are more or less sensitive to dairy. Medical tests and experts can help to evaluate whether you are lactose intolerant or allergic to milk proteins. One of the simplest procedures is to eliminate dairy from your diet for several weeks, as in the Rest and Repair Diet, then reintroduce milk and carefully monitor its effects on your body and mind.

CHAPTER 17

Wheat

Many gut health experts today advocate a wheat-free diet. The Gallup Poll estimates that one in five Americans is experimenting with gluten-free products and the number of people who avoid wheat and other grains containing gluten is continually rising.

Because of the work of Dr. Alessio Fasano (which we discussed in Chapter 10), we now know how wheat, and specifically gluten, can aggravate your gut lining. His research on celiac patients clearly shows how gluten causes tight junctions to open, allowing undigested food and bacterial byproducts into the bloodstream, leading to inflammation.

There is another group of people who are gluten sensitive but don't have celiac disease. They are called non-celiac gluten sensitivity patients.

Gluten isn't the only culprit in wheat that can cause inflammation. Wheat contains a family of proteins called ATIs, amylase-trypsin inhibitors. In plants, ATIs are useful proteins that help the development of seeds and protect the plant against certain parasites. When we consume ATIs in wheat, however, they can trigger chronic inflammation and worsen such conditions as asthma, rheumatoid arthritis, multiple sclerosis, and inflammatory bowel disease.

Civilization has thrived on wheat for millennia. Why is the consumption of modern wheat causing health problems? The wheat we eat today is very different from that of our ancestors. Modern wheat has been hybridized and significantly altered, both physically and chemically.

A fascinating YouTube debate between Dr. David Perlmutter and Dr. John Douillard considers these questions from different points of view. Dr. Perlmutter, as we know, advocates a wheat-free diet. Dr. Douillard is an Ayurveda expert and the author of the book *Eat Wheat*. Dr. Douillard says that the problem with wheat is poor digestion and the toxins that contaminate modern wheat. He admits that many people are not able to digest wheat, but he's against telling everybody to switch to a gluten-free diet. He advocates using Ayurvedic programs to improve digestion and detoxify the body. Dr. Perlmutter agrees that improving digestion and getting rid of toxins is good, but he strongly urges everyone to go on a gluten-free diet—for the simple reason that so many people have a problem digesting gluten.

Both Dr. Perlmutter and Dr. Douillard agree that one of the biggest problems is that modern wheat is sprayed with glyphosate (gly-fo-sate), the main ingredient in the herbicide Roundup. Glyphosate is primarily used on genetically modified crops but it's also used as a desiccant to help dry non-organic wheat crops before harvest. Dr. Perlmutter, Dr. Douillard, and other health experts believe that glyphosate is affecting your gluten sensitivity, and that the rise in gluten intolerance and celiac disease is due to the increased use of this chemical.

Glyphosate

In 2017, US farmers applied a remarkable 1.35 million metric tons of glyphosate to their crops. But there is controversy about the toxicity of glyphosate.

In March 2015, the World Health Organization's International Agency for Research on Cancer classified glyphosate as "probably carcinogenic in humans" (category 2A), based on epidemiological studies, animal studies, and in-vitro studies. It has been reported that even low doses of glyphosate-based herbicides can cause liver and kidney damage in animals.

In November 2015, however, the European Food Safety Authority approved glyphosate and concluded that "the substance is unlikely to be genotoxic (i.e. damaging to DNA) or to pose a carcinogenic threat to humans." In 2016, a joint meeting of the United Nation's Food and Agriculture Organization Panel of Experts on Pesticide Residues in Food and the Environment and the World Health Organization Core Assessment Group on Pesticide Residues again maintained that glyphosate was not harmful, saying that it was "unlikely to be genotoxic at anticipated dietary exposures."

Two of the most prominent scientists against glyphosate are Anthony Samsel, cited as an Independent Scientist and Consultant, and Dr. Stephanie Seneff, from the Computer Science and Artificial Intelligence Laboratory at MIT. In a series of five papers, they conclude that glyphosate can lead to the development of a wide range of chronic diseases. A number of other papers, however, have strongly refuted their hypothesis, and again we are left with disagreement.

What we do know is that glyphosate is present everywhere—in wheat, other foods, water, even in Ben and Jerry's ice cream (although none of their ingredients are sprayed with the herbicide). A recent paper measured glyphosate levels in a group of normal subjects living near San Diego over a period of several decades, and found that not only are glyphosate levels rising, they are reaching levels which should certainly be of concern to health officials.

The most consistent and common recommendation among gut health experts is to eat locally grown organic and non-GMO foods. We agree with this recommendation, and when you are on the Rest and Repair Diet it's important for you to stop eating wheat for 3 weeks, and avoid all produce sprayed with chemicals. After 3 weeks, you can then reintroduce wheat and evaluate how you feel.

CHAPTER 18

Probiotics and Prebiotics

Probiotics are friendly living bacteria. In 1907, Nobel Prize Laureate Ilya Ilyich Mechnikov promoted probiotics in yogurt as a way to maintain better health and slow the aging process. No one took him seriously at the time, but today well-controlled clinical trials show that probiotics improve a number of intestinal conditions, including irritable bowel syndrome.

Do probiotics actually reseed your gut back to its normal state?

No one knows. Remember, a capsule of probiotics usually contains between 7 to 10 friendly species of bacteria, while your gut has hundreds of different species. Think of it as sending a small group of well-bred private school children into a gang-ridden inner city and hoping that they will be a positive influence. In one recent study, which we mentioned earlier, when probiotics were given after antibiotics, they were only able to reseed the gut in about half the patients. In the other half, the probiotics may have actually stopped the growth of certain friendly bacteria.

REST AND REPAIR DIET

Probiotics are one of the hottest areas of research today, and even though science doesn't fully understand how or why they work, this is no passing health fad. The National Institutes of Health lists almost 1000 human clinical trials presently exploring the effectiveness of probiotics to treat a wide range of diseases including: fibromyalgia, obesity, gastrointestinal function, irritable bowel syndrome, anxiety, depression, asthma, type 2 diabetes mellitus, hyperlipidemia, alcoholic liver disease, hypertension, rheumatoid arthritis, bacterial vaginosis, diverticular disease, respiratory infections in children, atopic dermatitis, fatty liver, lactose intolerance, coronary artery disease, bipolar disorder, antibiotic-associated diarrhea, hypertriglyceridemia, HIV, cancer, and necrotizing enterocolitis in preterm infants with very low body weight.

How can you choose the right probiotic for your particular gut?

Some studies indicate that both the type and the number of friendly bacteria in a probiotic are critical for its success. Many companies insist that probiotics need a special coating to survive the acid of the stomach and the digestive enzymes in the small intestine. Others say that probiotics must always be refrigerated. And everyone advertises their probiotic as the best.

At docgut.com you will find a rating chart that evaluates probiotics according to:

- Clinical research studies

- Number of different types of probiotic bacteria

- Quantity of friendly bacteria

- Price

- Number of Amazon reviews for each probiotic

What are Prebiotics?

Prebiotics are types of dietary fiber that feed your friendly bacteria. Some of the most potent prebiotics include: asparagus, bananas, barley, oats, cocoa, burdock root, flaxseed, wheat bran, seaweed, Jerusalem artichoke, dandelion greens, garlic, leeks, onions, inulin, gum arabic, and chicory root.

Research shows that prebiotics have a number of beneficial effects: improving calcium and other mineral absorption, boosting the immune system, reducing colorectal cancer risk, improving symptoms in inflammatory bowel disease, and improving digestion and elimination. Research is currently being done to determine the potential beneficial effects of prebiotics for a wide number of diseases.

The Rest and Repair Diet recommends that you take probiotics and prebiotics (the herbal preparation triphala is considered a prebiotic). If you haven't already started, we suggest that you begin to take probiotics *after* the main 3-week period of the Rest and Repair Diet.

PART 4

Where Are We Going?

CHAPTER 19

The Future of Medicine

The ancients knew that all disease begins in the gut, but this knowledge was lost over time. Although the advent of drugs has proven to be a quick fix for some conditions, chronic diseases are increasing. *Instead of treating the symptoms of a disease, we need to treat the underlying causes.* We now know that the right diet and lifestyle can turn off certain destructive genes and turn on other beneficial genes.

Alzheimer's disease is one of the clearest examples of why medicine *must* change. Enormous sums of money have been spent by government agencies, pharmaceutical companies, and biotechnology firms to halt this disease, yet out of 244 experimental Alzheimer's drugs tested from 2000 to 2010, only one (memantine) was approved and its results are modest at best.

Until very recently, if you were diagnosed with Alzheimer's, there was almost nothing doctors could do for you. The situation has now changed. Preliminary research by Dr. Dale Bredesen shows an unprecedented success in reducing cognitive decline in early Alzheimer's patients through a special diet and changes in lifestyle.

Knowingly or unknowingly, most of us have repeatedly made poor choices in diet and lifestyle, and these choices, according to Dr. Bredesen, have resulted in specific genes being turned on, which eventually lead to Alzheimer's disease.

The Bredesen approach includes 36 different tests, so it's not a trivial undertaking and requires a qualified doctor's assistance. Dr. Bredesen's program recommends a special diet and numerous changes in lifestyle, but patients can begin with simple changes, such as improving their gut health and learning to meditate.

It is important for individuals to be proactive about their health and take steps to prevent chronic diseases like Alzheimer's. The key is in integrating ancient and modern health practices, and providing additional training to help doctors and health coaches improve their patient's mind/body health. The microbiome is the missing link that unifies your understanding of both ancient and modern concepts and offers new hope for the future of medicine.

The Rest and Repair Diet is an important first step, which easily integrates modern medicine with the ancient knowledge of Ayurveda. By taking responsibility for your own health, and using the diet and lifestyle recommendations of the Rest and Repair Diet, you have already begun your journey to a healthier, more resilient state of mind and body.

CHAPTER 20

Health Coaching

You might start the Rest and Repair Diet with all good intentions and then, part way through, a craving (or two or three) arises. Suddenly you're having an agonizingly hard time staying on the diet.

One of the most challenging parts of any diet program is compliance—in other words, *sticking to it*. Compliance is especially tough when you are trying to stop eating an addictive food like sugar.

It's a lot easier if you invite a friend or acquaintance who is also on the diet, to be your buddy or partner. During the main 3 weeks, especially, it's good to check in with your buddy for a few minutes every day. Mutual support and a little encouragement is a very good thing. On this diet, your buddy acts as a sort of "health coach" for you.

There are different definitions of the term "health coach," and also different levels of experience and expertise. A properly trained coach will ask questions that allow you to set realistic goals, and help you find ways of checking in with yourself to make sure that you're accomplishing those goals.

Health coaches are the future of modern medicine. We all know that a better diet, more exercise, a good sleep routine, and the practice of meditation, are ways to avoid chronic disease. The problem is that most of us would rather take a pill than make the effort to change our lifestyle habits, especially when it comes to diet.

During your Self Discovery Lifestyle program, the most ideal situation would be for you to work with an Ayurvedic health coach who is trained and certified in the Rest and Repair Diet (see Appendix 2), and who can offer you a deeper level of education about which foods are best for your individual constitution. An Ayurveda health coach can also help you personalize lifestyle programs in areas such as exercise, yoga, sleep, and meditation.

Awareness is the key to making positive changes in your life. It's not easy to give up ingrained habits or cravings, and a good coach can help you to become self-sufficient in achieving your goals. The ultimate goal of the Rest and Repair Diet is for you to *become your own health coach.*

Health Coaching

PART 5

Ayurveda and Integrative Medicine for All Ages

CHAPTER 21

The Different Gut/Brain Natures

In Chapter 6, we describe how Ayurveda defines your mind and body in terms of three main characteristics, or doshas, called Vata, Pitta, and Kapha. Each person is a unique combination of these three fundamental tendencies. We use the more modern term Gut/Brain Nature, rather than doshas, in order to emphasize the importance of the gut-brain axis to your health. Including combinations, there are seven possible Gut/Brain Natures, and each is described in detail below. We also include the different foods recommended by Ayurveda for each Gut/Brain Nature. If you don't know your Gut/Brain Nature, go to our website at docgut. com and take the quiz to discover your individual combination.

Vata or V Gut/Brain Nature

V Digestion

Those of you with a Vata or V Gut/Brain Nature have wide swings in your appetite and digestive power, strong at one moment, weak at another. You're a "snacker," who enjoys and actually benefits from eating several small nutritious meals throughout the day. It is important for you to eat in a quiet environment, away from distractions.

When your V Gut is balanced, your digestion is good. When you're out of balance, however, you may experience symptoms of constipation, indigestion, and gas.

You will greatly benefit from a good routine that helps keep your feet planted firmly on mother earth.

Your V Watchwords are STAY GROUNDED!

The following recommendations will help your digestion and metabolism:

- Always sit down when eating

- Eat in a settled environment

- Start the day with a warm breakfast

- Lunch should be the biggest meal of the day. Snack with roasted nuts and seeds (raw nuts are more difficult for you to digest)

- Avoid cold drinks while eating, since the cold will impair digestion

- Sip hot water during the day and if possible carry a small thermos and drink a cup every hour or two

Ideal Foods for Vata

The general guideline is that sweet, sour, salty, heavy, oily, and hot foods are best for Vatas. Pungent, bitter, astringent, light, dry, and cold foods are not good. Warm heavy foods are easier to digest and assimilate. They also help to sooth and balance your Vata. An ideal breakfast for a V Gut is cooked cereal with roasted nuts and a little fruit (if gluten intolerant, use an appropriate non-gluten grain). Avoid or reduce stimulants like coffee, tea, and other caffeine-laden beverages. Cool it on the alcohol.

1. **Best veggies:** asparagus, beets, cucumbers, green beans, okra, radishes, sweet potatoes, turnips, carrots, and artichokes. Other vegetables may be eaten in moderation if cooked in ghee (clarified butter) or extra-virgin olive oil. Avoid or reduce cabbage, cauliflower, Brussels sprouts, or bean sprouts. No raw vegetables except for small leafy salads.

2. **Best spices:** anise, basil, cardamom, cilantro, cinnamon, clove, cumin, fennel, fenugreek, ginger, licorice root, marjoram, nutmeg, oregano, salt, mustard seed, sage, tarragon, thyme and black pepper. Minimize or eliminate all bitter, pungent, and astringent spices.

3. **Any organic dairy product** is highly recommended. Milk is easier for Vatas to digest when heated (unless you are lactose intolerant!). The warmth will also help to balance your Vata. Instead of skim milk, dilute whole milk with purified water. If sleep is a problem, bring a cup of whole milk to a boil 4 times, then add cardamom, cinnamon, nutmeg, and coconut sugar to taste. Drink while nicely warm, not hot. (If milk clogs you up overnight add a *little* powdered ginger. Too much can be over-stimulating and keep you up, or cause a stomach ache.)

4. **Favor rice, wheat** (if you can tolerate gluten), and cooked oats. And reduce your consumption of corn (fresh corn on the cob in season is great), millet, barley, buckwheat, and rye.

5. **Favor sweet, well-ripened fruits** such as apricots, plums, berries, melons, papayas, peaches, cherries, nectarines, and bananas. Also good are dates, figs, pineapples, and mangoes. If you have digestive problems, fruits are best eaten lightly stewed or sautéed. Avocados (technically a fruit) are very good for Vatas.

6. All oils should be consumed frequently and generously. Clarified butter (ghee), and olive oil are especially good for Vata.

7. **All sweeteners** are acceptable. Favor coconut sugar. Avoid artificial sweeteners.

8. All nuts and seeds are good, especially almonds (soaking them overnight and then roasting is best).

9. Vata types are usually very sensitive to gas-producing foods such as beans so they should be avoided.

10. **Beans** such as chickpeas, mung beans, and tofu, however, are fine in small amounts.

11. For non-vegetarians, favor fresh, organic chicken, turkey, fish, and eggs. Reduce or eliminate the consumption of red meat and pork.

12. **Vata Tea** helps to balance and restore your Vata Nature (see Appendix 1).

13. **Vata Spice** mix (see Appendix 1)

V Physical Characteristics

V Gut/Brain natures tend to be thinner, especially at a younger age, and have a hard time gaining weight. You generally move fast, think fast, and have bursts of energy. You are always the one who wants to turn up the heat and dislikes being in the wind. It's critical for Vatas to stay warm in all seasons. Layering is a good way to maintain body temperature because clothing can be removed or added as needed. Don't go out in cold or windy weather unless properly dressed. Hats are a must!

You tend towards dryness both inside and out. It's not enough to just moisturize your skin, you also need to moisturize your insides by adding healthy organic oils to your diet. Good choices are clarified butter (ghee), olive oil, avocado oil, and coconut oil.

To moisturize your skin, use a rich warm oil (cured and heated sesame oil is traditionally recommended for Vatas) or a penetrating organic moisturizer from head to toe after your morning shower. Especially in winter, you need to apply oils to any part of your body exposed to the elements (including indoor heating).

Vatas need to keep well hydrated by sipping at least 6 cups of hot water every day. All your tissues, especially hair and skin, will benefit!

V Mental and Emotional Behavior

Your V Gut/Brain emotions are constantly changing. You are creative and have a great imagination. You're quick to learn, quick to forget, and particularly good at verbal skills and the arts. You usually enjoy talking. Your mind is constantly active. Your attention moves rapidly from one topic to another, so you must do what you can to stay balanced and focused.

You are sensitive to sensory inputs, and need to protect yourself from excess stimulation and tiredness. You can be very active and happy (balanced) for quite some time, then suddenly become unfocused and anxious (imbalanced). You should avoid caffeine after 10 in the morning because it aggravates your Vata mind. You already have irregular sleep habits and excitement at night can lead to insomnia.

V Imbalances and General Recommendations

V Causes of Imbalance

- Overstimulation
- Too many choices
- Overexertion
- Negative emotions
- Irregular routine
- Stressful situations
- Exposure to cold and/or windy weather
- Unpleasant interactions
- Excessive travel

V Results of Imbalance

- Hyperactivity
- Restlessness
- Distraction
- Nervousness
- Heightened emotions
- Forgetfulness
- Anxiousness
- Poor digestion
- Fearfulness
- Constipation
- Loneliness
- Irregular appetite
- Rapid mood changes
- Inability to focus

V Recommendations

- Establish and maintain a daily routine
- Have healthy snacks
- Protect from cold, windy weather
- Avoid video games at night
- Reduce excessive stimulation
- Maintain a fixed bedtime routine
- Make plans and goals

- Minimize the number of choices
- Guard against fatigue
- Engage in creative activities
- Take naps to recharge physically and emotionally

Remember:

- **Stay Grounded**

- **Stay Warm**

- **Stay Rested**

- **Stick To A Good Routine**

Pitta or P Gut/Brain Nature

P Digestion

The essence of the Pitta or P Gut/Brain Nature is a powerful digestive fire. Your P Gut is programmed to produce a strong appetite, which needs to be fed at particular times during the day.

When your P Gut is balanced, your digestion is highly efficient. The downside is that you need to eat on time. If not, you can become demanding and irritable—even to the point of anger. When you are out of balance, you can also experience hyperacidity.

Your P Watchwords are EAT ON TIME!

The following recommendations will help your digestion and metabolism:

- Eat good size meals on time

- Start the day with cooked fruit, followed by cereal

- Never skip meals—eat at least every 3 hours

- Delaying meals can cause excess acidity and crankiness— eat all meals on time

- Eat your largest meal at lunch when digestion is strongest

- Eat a lighter meal for dinner

- Avoid hot spices like peppers and chilies—spicy foods aggravate a P gut and overheat both mind and body

- Favor cooling foods and liquids

- Don't rush through your meal—enjoy your food and the company around you

- Heartburn or upset stomach results if you eat too quickly

- Chew food well—most P Gut people eat much too fast

- Keep hydrated—if you are overheated, drink more fluids

- Snack on sweet juicy fruits: ripe pears, sweet grapes, and fully ripe mangoes.

Ideal Foods for Pitta Types

The general guideline is: sweet, bitter, astringent, cold, heavy, and dry foods are best for Pittas. Pungent, sour, salty, and hot foods can create an imbalance.

1. **Best veggies:** asparagus, potatoes, sweet potatoes, leafy greens, broccoli, cauliflower, celery, okra, lettuce, green beans, peas, and zucchini. Also good are Brussels sprouts, cabbage, cucumbers, mushrooms, sprouts, and sweet peppers. Avoid or reduce tomatoes, hot peppers, onions, garlic, and hot radishes.

2. **All sweeteners** are okay in moderation, except for molasses and honey, which are heating to the system.

3. **Dairy** is helpful in balancing Pitta. Favor butter, ghee, milk, and ice cream. Since the sour taste can increase Pitta, sour or fermented products such as yogurt, sour cream, and cheese should be eaten sparingly. Lassi is considered to be different from yogurt even though it is made from yogurt, and has a balancing effect on Pitta.

4. **Organic grains such as wheat, rice, barley, and oats** are good. Reduce consumption of corn, rye, millet, and brown rice.

5. **Sweet and ripe fruits** like apples, grapes, melons, cherries, coconuts, avocados, mangoes, pineapples, figs, oranges, and plums are recommended. Also prunes, raisins, and dried figs are fine. Reduce or eliminate sour fruits such as grapefruit, cranberries, lemons, and persimmons.

6. Pitta types need **seasonings that are soothing and cooling.** These include coriander, cilantro, cardamom, and saffron. Turmeric, dill, fennel, and mint are also fine. Spices such as ginger, black pepper, fenugreek, clove, salt, and mustard seed may be used sparingly. Completely *avoid* pungent hot spices such as chili peppers and cayenne.

7. **Most nuts** increase Pitta; however, roasted pumpkin seeds and sunflower seeds are all right.

8. **Favor coconut, olive, and sunflower oils.** Avoid or reduce almond, corn, safflower, and sesame oils.

9. **Favor mung beans and chickpeas.** Fresh tofu and other soy products are all right.

10. For non-vegetarians, organic free-range chicken and turkey are preferable. Red meat, pork, and seafood increase Pitta and should be avoided.

11. **Pitta Tea** helps to balance and restore your Pitta Nature (see Appendix 1).

12. **Pitta Spice** mix (see Appendix 1)

P Physical Characteristics

You are usually strong and resilient, full of energy, and rarely get sick.

But you probably rely heavily on your body to push through the early stages of illness rather than paying attention to your need for rest. This, of course, can lead to exhaustion. Your Achilles heel is that you are highly vulnerable to becoming imbalanced if you don't eat on time or become over-heated—which can occur very quickly.

You tend to have a competitive nature—useful in many situations, but which you need to keep in a positive direction. It takes good physical activity to absorb your enormous energy. Many Pitta people are natural athletes

You overheat easily, so it's very important to make sure to drink lots of water and stay in the shade or air conditioning as much as possible during hot weather. Dress in lightweight, breathable clothing made from natural fibers, wear a hat, and use a good sunscreen (see recommendations by the Environmental Working Group at ewg.com) when heading outdoors.

P Mental and Emotional Behavior

You are strong willed and your intellect is sharp. It is easy for you to be highly focused and on-task when solving problems. You are good at getting things done and getting them done on time.

You have a responsive and highly dynamic temperament with strong emotions and may stop at nothing to complete a task or achieve your goals. You enjoy being around people and might be a good leader. So it's very important to remember to balance your drive by staying cool, calm, and compassionate, especially during challenging situations. Your impulse is to forge ahead. It is better to force yourself to relax a little, rather than moving at warp speed, dragging everyone else behind.

In your balanced state, you are energetic and purposeful. In an imbalanced state, you can become controlling, demanding, and irritable, and you may lose your temper, even become aggressive.

You need to moderate or avoid stimulants such as coffee and other substances that increase your internal fire, even though you probably enjoy the rush. Meditating, swimming, listening to relaxing music and drinking cool liquids help to soothe your fiery nature and keep your mood lighthearted.

P Imbalances and General Recommendations

P Causes of Imbalance

- Overheating
- Not eating on time
- Hot spices such as chilies
- Stimulating TV, video games
- Not enough cool liquids
- Overly competitive situations
- Negative emotions

P Results of Imbalance

- Irritability
- Intense hunger
- Impatience
- Excessive thirst
- Anger
- Sensitivity to spicy and/or fried foods
- Being critical
- Indigestion and/or heartburn
- Aggression or hostility
- Excessive perspiration
- Jealousy
- Hot temper
- Obsessive-compulsive behaviors

P Recommendations

- Eat on time, especially lunch
- Exercise regularly but don't overdo it
- Swimming and water sports to cool and balance
- Prevent overheating
- Keep the air conditioner running
- Drink plenty of cooling liquids
- Avoid spicy foods

Remember:

- **Eat On Time**

- **Engage In Physical Activity Every Day**

- **Be Careful Not To Overheat In Any Season**

- **Drink Lots Of Water!**

Kapha or K Gut/Brain Nature

K Digestion

With a Kapha or K Gut/Brain Nature, digestion is steady and you can even miss a meal and be fine. You love food but you need to eat smaller amounts since you have a slower metabolism. Of the three main types, you tend to drink the least amount of water.

When your K Gut is balanced, your digestion works well. When out of balance, you can gain weight very easily, so you need to be careful not to overeat.

Your K Watchwords are MOVE IT!

The following recommendations will help your digestion and metabolism:

- Start the day with a light breakfast

- Eat your largest meal at lunch when digestive fire is strongest (other times it's low)

- Eat a small warm meal in the evening

- Optimize your metabolism by sipping hot water throughout the day

- Too much dairy, fried foods, or fatty meats are not good for your digestion

- Excess carbs and fat intake slows both your digestion and metabolism and will definitely add weight

- Get lots of physical activity

Ideal Foods for Kapha

The general guideline is that pungent, bitter, astringent, light, hot, and dry foods are best for Kaphas. Sweet, sour, salty, heavy, oily, and cold foods are not recommended.

1. **Most vegetables** are good for you, including asparagus, beets, broccoli, Brussels sprouts, cabbage, carrots, cauliflower, celery, eggplants, leafy greens, lettuce, mushrooms, okra, onions, peas, peppers, pumpkins, potatoes, radishes, spinach, and sprouts. Reduce the consumption of such vegetables as sweet potatoes, tomatoes, cucumbers, and zucchini.

2. **Favor skim milk.** In general, reduce dairy intake, which tends to increase Kapha. You can, however, add small amounts of ghee, whole milk, and eggs to the menu. Reduce or avoid butter, cheese, cream, yogurt, and buttermilk.

3. **Honey** (raw, unheated, and organic) is the only sweetener that helps balance Kapha. Avoid all others.

4. **Favor grains such as barley, corn, millet, buckwheat, and rye.** Reduce intake of oats, rice, and wheat.

5. **Beans of all types** are good for Kaphas, except soybeans, tofu products, and kidney beans.

6. **Fruits such as apples, apricots, cranberries, pears, persimmons, and pomegranates** are good. Avoid or reduce fruits like avocados, bananas, pineapples, oranges, peaches, coconuts, melons, dates, figs, grapefruit, grapes, mangoes, papayas, and plums.

7. **All spices except salt** are good for Kapha. Pungent spices like ginger, pepper, and mustard seed are excellent for your digestion. Reduce salt.

8. **Reduce the intake of all nuts** and seeds, except for pumpkin seeds and sunflower seeds,

9. Use **small amounts** of extra-virgin olive oil, ghee, almond oil, corn oil, sunflower oil, or safflower oil.

10. For non-vegetarians, favor fresh, organic free-range chicken and turkey. Small amounts of eggs are okay.

11. Limit or eliminate the consumption of red meat, pork, and seafood.

12. **Kapha Tea** helps to balance and restore your Kapha Nature (see Appendix 1).

13. **Kapha Spice** mix (see Appendix 1)

K Physical Characteristics

Even at an early age, you showed physical strength and endurance. You often have a solid or heavy body frame, and tend to gain weight more easily than other types. Of the three primary natures, you are the least sensitive to weather, but you don't do well in either cold and damp or warm and humid conditions.

Sleep is your best friend. You fall asleep easily and have a far better chance of staying asleep throughout the night than others. But it may be hard to wake up in the morning. Plan ahead to allow yourself extra time to get dressed and ready for work or appointments.

When you are out of balance, you can become lethargic, gain weight, or withdraw, and you may become depressed.

K Mental and Emotional Behavior

You are stable, patient, and easy going, and are rarely disturbed by changes in your environment. You tend to be methodical and slow when learning new things, but once you learn something you don't forget it! You often take extra time making decisions because you want to be thorough.

Your most outstanding characteristic is the quality of steadiness—but this steadiness can sometimes slow you down, cause you to be attached to routines, and become too rigid. It's good to introduce extra stimulation and variety in your life to help you become more flexible and motivated.

When you are out of balance, you can become lethargic, stubborn, depressed, and withdrawn. You would rather stay in bed watching TV and eating ice cream. You need to avoid dwelling on situations that you can't change, and focus on your bright future. It's important for you to be as optimistic and light as possible.

K Imbalances And General Recommendations

K Causes of Imbalance

- Excessive sleep
- Overeating
- Too little activity
- Exposure to hot, humid weather
- Lack of mental stimulation
- Exposure to cold, damp weather
- Lack of regular exercise

K Results of Imbalance

- Stubbornness
- Sadness
- Depression
- Withdrawal
- Lethargy
- Excess mucus
- Laziness
- Weight gain

K Recommendations

- Keep mentally and physically stimulated
- Try a dehumidifier
- If it's damp and cold, have warm drinks
- Include exercise in your routine
- Try not to overeat; light meals are best
- Volunteering can build nurturing bonds
- Welcome new relationships—get out and meet people
- Be easy about adapting to change

Remember:

- **Be Active**

- **Allow Extra Time To Do Everything**

- **Stay Challenged—Learn New Things**

- **Motivation Is Everything!**

Combination Natures

VP (PV) Gut/Brain Nature

VP Digestion

With your Vata Pitta Nature (which is virtually the same as the Pitta Vata Nature) your digestion is strong but variable, and your appetite is good. Because you are part V Gut, you may, however, be a picky (or discriminating!) eater with strong preferences. You can be hungry one minute and not the next. And because you are part P Gut, you need ample meals to sustain your physical and mental activity. As a combination type, you have a more balanced appetite than people with a pure V or a pure P Gut.

When you're in balance, you rarely have digestive problems. When you're out of balance, your digestive issues can range from weak digestion to hyperactivity.

Your VP Watchwords are REST, STAY COOL, and EAT ON TIME!

The following recommendations will help your digestion and metabolism:

- Start the day with a warm, nutritious breakfast

- Always sit when eating and eat in a settled environment

- Have a hot nourishing lunch as close to mid-day as possible. It should be your biggest meal of the day

- Avoid spicy food because it will aggravate the P Gut part of your digestive system

- Snack on fruit, roasted nuts and seeds

- Enjoy a small dinner at the end of the day

- Sit quietly for a few minutes after eating—don't rush into activity

- Enjoy cool drinks on warm days

Ideal Food for Vata/Pitta

Determining the best diet for a mixed Gut/Brain Nature is tricky. Foods that are good for one of your types may not be so good for the other. This is one of the reasons we recommend that you consult a well-trained Gut/Brain or Ayurvedic practitioner. He or she will be better able to make recommendations for your personal situation, based not only on your nature, but also on any imbalances.

Generally, experts say that people with mixed natures should choose the foods they like best from the "Favor" columns. Experiment to see what works best for you.

VP Physical Characteristics

As a VP, you have lots of energy and may be both agile and graceful, but you are more likely to be a sprinter rather than a long distance runner. When you are in good balance, you draw energy from your P qualities. When you are out of balance, your V qualities can cause you to become overstimulated and exhausted. This duality gives you reasonably strong but variable energy.

If you listen to your body, you'll be able to maintain a more optimum Gut/Brain level of functioning and prevent serious conditions caused by extreme or long-term imbalances.

VP Mental and Emotional Behavior

You are creative and artistic and have a good intellect and the ability to learn quickly. Your V qualities make you emotionally sensitive. Your P emotions give you drive, passion, and enjoyment of the feeling of being in control. It's more important (and it will make your life easier) to respect and nurture your relationships, rather than to be "right."

Your two main characteristics can either complement OR aggravate each other. So you can quickly jump between being a fountain of new ideas to laser-like, almost obsessive focus on details, depending on which characteristic is dominant or out of balance. It's important to correct any imbalance as it arises, and before it can cause both V and P go out of balance.

When your two sides work together, this enables you to be inspirational, courageous, and motivated. When these powerful qualities go out of balance, however, they can quickly lead to anxiety, anger, and burnout. It's like wind on a wildfire, which causes the flames to burn hotter and spread quickly.

Before making an important decision, allow problems to sit quietly in your great brain overnight. Don't jump to conclusions. Decisions are likely to come more easily and produce better results when you are rested.

VP Imbalances and General Recommendations

You need to look at your problems in the context of your dual nature. What follows are the causes and signs of imbalances which you might experience, and general recommendations for both of your Gut/Brain Natures.

V Causes of Imbalance

- Overstimulation
- Too many choices
- Overexertion
- Negative emotions
- Irregular routine
- Stressful situations
- Exposure to cold and/or windy weather
- Unpleasant interactions
- Excessive travel

V Results of Imbalance

- Hyperactivity
- Restlessness
- Distraction
- Nervousness
- Heightened emotions
- Forgetfulness
- Anxiousness
- Poor digestion

- Fearfulness
- Constipation
- Loneliness

- Irregular appetite
- Rapid mood changes
- Inability to focus

V Recommendations

- Establish and maintain a daily routine
- Have healthy snacks
- Protect from cold, windy weather
- Avoid video games at night
- Reduce excessive stimulation

- Maintain a fixed bedtime routine
- Make plans and goals
- Minimize the number of choices
- Guard against fatigue
- Engage in creative activities
- Take naps to recharge physically and emotionally

P Causes of Imbalance

- Overheating
- Not eating on time
- Hot spices such as chilies
- Stimulating TV, video games

- Not enough cool liquids
- Overly competitive situations
- Negative emotions

P Results of Imbalance

- Irritability
- Intense hunger
- Impatience
- Excessive thirst

- Anger
- Sensitivity to spicy and/or fried foods
- Being critical

- Indigestion and/ or heartburn
- Aggression or hostility
- Excessive perspiration
- Jealousy
- Hot temper
- Obsessive-compulsive behaviors

P Recommendations

- Eat on time, especially lunch
- Exercise regularly but don't overdo it
- Swimming and water sports to cool and balance
- Prevent overheating
- Keep the air conditioner running
- Drink plenty of cooling liquids
- Avoid spicy foods

Remember:

- **Maintain A Supportive Daily Routine**

- **Get Extra Rest**

- **Eat On Time**

- **Stay Hydrated!**

VK (KV) Gut/Brain Nature

VK Digestion

With your Vata Kapha Nature (virtually the same as Kapha Vata), your digestion is generally strong and steady, and you enjoy an occasional snack. You're a combination of V, which makes you a grazer with a constantly changing appetite, and K, which makes you love to eat. Fortunately, V and K complement each other *when they are in balance*. So, you enjoy food, but don't gain as much weight as pure K types.

When you are out of balance, your digestion slows down and you become more sensitive to what you eat.

Your VK Watchwords are GROUND YOURSELF and MOVE IT!

The following recommendations will help your digestion and metabolism:

- Start the day with a warm nourishing breakfast

- Always sit to eat

- Eat in a happy, peaceful atmosphere without distractions like TV, games, and cell phones

- Do not skip meals

- Make a hot, filling lunch your largest meal of the day

- Have a light but grounding meal for dinner

- A meal plan will help keep your digestion and metabolism as optimal as possible

- Enjoy exercise every day

- Good company will keep you happy and engaged and help your digestion

Ideal Food for Vata/Kapha

Determining the best diet for a mixed Gut/Brain Nature is tricky. Foods that are good for one of your types may not be so good for the other. This is one of the reasons we recommend that you consult a well-trained Gut/Brain or Ayurvedic practitioner. He or she will be better able to make recommendations for your personal situation, based not only on your nature, but also on any imbalances.

Generally, experts say that people with mixed natures should choose the foods they like best from the "Favor" columns. Experiment to see what works best for you.

VK Physical Characteristics

You are an interesting combination of opposites. Your V Nature is light and airy, while your K Nature is heavy and earthy.

You may be tall and either well built or stout, but with delicate features. You're prone to gaining weight due to your K's slow and sometime variable metabolism. Your weight can be evenly distributed over your whole body, or can lodge in certain areas like hips, thighs, or buttocks.

When balanced, you are healthy and have good physical stamina. When you are out of balance you're prone to frequent colds and respiratory problems. An imbalance of Vata will always push your Kapha out of balance, so you need to address imbalances as soon as you become aware of them. You don't do well in cold or damp weather, so it's important to stay warm.

VK Mental and Emotional Behavior

The VK combination gives rise to individuals who have a wide range of emotions. You are quick, inspiring, and full of new ideas, but at the same time stable, well liked, and methodical. You can be both grounded and sensitive. One side of you is in motion, while the other is steady and constant.

When you're imbalanced, you tend to be spacey, withdrawn, or even depressed. You can obsess on issues, and become attached and anxious. It's especially good for you to have enjoyable social outings and stay rested, energized, and happy in order to improve every aspect of your mind, body, and emotions.

VK Imbalances and General Recommendations

You need to look at your problems in the context of your dual nature. What follows are the causes and signs of imbalances which you might experience, and general recommendations for both of your Gut/Brain Natures.

V Causes of Imbalance

- Overstimulation
- Too many choices
- Overexertion
- Negative emotions
- Irregular routine
- Stressful situations
- Exposure to cold and/or windy weather
- Unpleasant interactions
- Excessive travel

V Results of Imbalance

- Hyperactivity
- Restlessness
- Distraction
- Nervousness
- Heightened emotions
- Forgetfulness
- Anxiousness
- Poor digestion
- Fearfulness
- Constipation
- Loneliness
- Irregular appetite
- Rapid mood changes
- Inability to focus

V Recommendations

- Establish and maintain a daily routine
- Have healthy snacks
- Protect from cold, windy weather
- Avoid video games at night
- Reduce excessive stimulation
- Maintain a fixed bedtime routine

- Make plans and goals
- Minimize the number of choices
- Guard against fatigue
- Engage in creative activities
- Take naps to recharge physically and emotionally

K Causes of Imbalance

- Excessive sleep
- Overeating
- Too little activity
- Exposure to hot, humid weather
- Lack of mental stimulation
- Exposure to cold, damp weather
- Lack of regular exercise

K Results of Imbalance

- Stubbornness
- Sadness
- Depression
- Withdrawal
- Lethargy
- Excess mucus
- Laziness
- Weight gain

K Recommendations

- Keep mentally and physically stimulated
- Try a dehumidifier
- If it's damp and cold, have warm drinks
- Include exercise in your routine
- Try not to overeat; light meals are best
- Volunteering can build nurturing bonds
- Welcome new relationships—get out and meet people

- Be easy about adapting to change

Remember:

- **Follow A Good Routine (For Your V Nature)**

- **Occasionally Spice Your Routine Up With Variety (For Your K Nature)**

- **In Cold Weather, Keep Toasty With Multiple Layers**

PK (KP) Gut/Brain Nature

PK Digestion

With your Pitta Kapha Nature (which is virtually the same as Kapha Pitta), your digestion and appetite are both strong. Anyone with a P Gut has a good appetite. If you have a PK Gut, you will have an even better appetite. You like to eat lots of food and can generally digest it easily. However, because you are part K Gut, your metabolism can slow down at times and you may have a hard time digesting greasy foods. Although it's easy for you to gain a few extra pounds, you can usually lose them without much effort.

When you are in balance, you rarely have digestive problems. When out of balance, beware of slower digestion and hyperacidity.

Your PK Watchwords are EAT ON TIME! and MOVE IT!

The following recommendations will help your digestion and metabolism:

- Start the day with cooked fruit—apples are a great breakfast food

- In a pinch, try applesauce with cinnamon and a few nuts, followed by cereal for breakfast

- Avoid spicy food that can aggravate your P Gut Nature

- Stay well hydrated

- Have cool drinks on warm days

- Don't skip meals

- Don't wait to eat until ravenously hungry

- Snack on ripe fruit, roasted seeds and nuts when hungry

- Have a hot, substantial meal at lunch and a lighter meal at dinner

- Food cravings increase when you are emotionally upset

- Exercise regularly to lose extra weight and maintain physical and emotional balance

Ideal Food for Pitta/Kapha

Determining the best diet for a mixed Gut/Brain Nature is tricky. Foods that are good for one of your types may not be so good for the other. This is one of the reasons we recommend that you consult a well-trained Gut/Brain or Ayurvedic practitioner. He or she will be better able to make recommendations for your personal situation, based not only on your nature, but also on any imbalances.

Generally, experts say that people with mixed natures should choose the foods they like best from the "Favor" columns. Experiment to see what works best for you.

PK Physical Characteristics

You have the hot, transformative qualities of a P Nature plus the cool, stable qualities of a K Nature. If you don't stay in balance you can boil over. You are generally large and strong. You may not be the star of the team, but you have the constitution to be a good player.

You really need to exercise daily. If you become a couch potato, you can expect to add extra pounds. Fortunately, you can also lose them easily. You have good stamina in activity, but you have to be careful not to get overheated.

You rarely enjoy cold, damp conditions and need to be careful in late spring, summer, and early fall, especially if it's hot and humid. You can easily heat up and become exhausted and irritable. In the summer, you need to be alert for ways to cool down. From late winter to late spring it's easy for you to become a little lazy.

Work out imbalances as soon as possible to prevent them from becoming deeper or chronic, before they manifest as illness.

PK Mental and Emotional Behavior

You tend to be strong, sturdy, content, and easy going. Your drive is steadied by your calm, easy going nature. Imbalances can cause impatience, anger, and lethargy. You can also become argumentative, stubborn, and withdrawn. It's important for you, particularly, to maintain healthy family relationships and friendships to stay in good balance.

In the heat of the moment you may not think problems through completely. And if decisions backfire, you can be prone to useless regret. It's important for you to spend more time listening and less time making assumptions and running scenarios in your head.

PK Imbalances and General Recommendations

You need to look at your problems in the context of your dual nature. What follows are the causes and signs of imbalances that you might experience, and general recommendations for your dual Gut/Brain nature.

P Causes of Imbalance

- Overheating
- Not eating on time
- Hot spices such as chilies
- Stimulating TV, video games
- Not enough cool liquids
- Overly competitive situations
- Negative emotions

P Results of Imbalance

- Irritability
- Intense hunger
- Impatience
- Excessive thirst
- Anger
- Sensitivity to spicy and/or fried foods
- Being critical
- Indigestion and/ or heartburn
- Aggression or hostility
- Excessive perspiration
- Jealousy
- Hot temper
- Obsessive-compulsive behaviors

P Recommendations

- Eat on time, especially lunch
- Exercise regularly but don't overdo it
- Swimming and water sports to cool and balance

- Prevent overheating
- Keep the air conditioner running
- Drink plenty of cooling liquids
- Avoid spicy foods

K Causes of Imbalance

- Excessive sleep
- Overeating
- Too little activity
- Exposure to hot, humid weather
- Lack of mental stimulation
- Exposure to cold, damp weather
- Lack of regular exercise

K Results of Imbalance

- Stubbornness
- Sadness
- Depression
- Withdrawal
- Lethargy
- Excess mucus
- Laziness
- Weight gain

K Recommendations

- Keep mentally and physically stimulated
- Try a dehumidifier
- If it's damp and cold, have warm drinks
- Include exercise in your routine
- Try not to overeat; light meals are best
- Volunteering can build nurturing bonds
- Welcome new relationships—get out and meet people
- Be easy about adapting to change

Remember:

- **Welcome New Experiences And Outings**

- **Move: You Need Physical Exercise Every Day**

- **Daily Meditation And Yoga Keep You Balanced**

VPK Gut/Brain or Tri Nature

VPK Digestion

With your Vata/Pitta/Kapha Nature, your appetite and digestion is good. Since you have a stronger constitution than others, you can eat almost any kind of food and rarely experience excessive hunger or thirst. But because your symptoms are usually mild and somewhat veiled, it's hard to pinpoint how and when you go out of balance. You really need to learn to listen to your body.

Your VPK Watchwords are LISTEN TO YOUR BODY and BE AWARE OF YOUR TENDENCIES

The following recommendations will help your digestion and metabolism:

- Sit when eating and try not to skip meals

- Your largest meal should be lunch

- Eat moderately and regularly

- Planning balanced meals will help to keep your digestion and metabolism as optimal as possible

- Enjoy meditation and exercise every day

Ideal Food for Vata/Pitta/Kapha

Determining the best diet for a mixed Gut/Brain Nature is tricky. Foods that are good for one of your types may not be so good for the other. This is one of the reasons we recommend that you consult a well-trained Gut/Brain or Ayurvedic practitioner. He or she will be better able to make recommendations for your personal situation, based not only on your nature, but also on any imbalances.

Generally, experts say that people with mixed natures should choose the foods they like best from the "Favor" columns. Experiment to see what works best for you.

VPK Physical Characteristics

You are a relatively rare mixture of the three types, and show the best qualities of each. Physically strong with a moderate build, you are usually in good health. If you can stay in balance, you may avoid most seasonal illnesses, experiencing only mild to moderate symptoms during each season (like dry skin in the winter, a bit of lethargy in the spring, or mild heat intolerance in the summer).

Life becomes complicated when one or more of your Gut characteristics goes out of balance and it can be tricky to regain it. Especially as it may not be clear which nature was first to go out of balance. The best advice is to treat imbalances in the following order: 1) start with balancing Vata; 2) go on to balance Pitta; and 3) finally, address your Kapha. Keep in mind that it takes your

VPK constitution longer to go out of balance, but also longer to come back into balance than other natures.

VPK Mental and Emotional Behavior

You are creative, motivated, steady, and good natured. When balanced, you're in tune with your body and emotions and are quite intuitive. Because of your amazing range of emotions - from highly passionate to steady and patient—it may be harder for you to identify when you are emotionally imbalanced. The first signs of imbalance can be mild anxiety, irritability, or even depression. Stay alert to when something isn't quite right.

Although you have an easier time remaining in good balance compared to other types, imbalances still occur and can take longer to correct.

VPK Imbalances and General Recommendations

You need to look at your problems in the context of your dual nature. What follows are the causes and signs of imbalances, which you might experience, and general recommendations for all 3 of your Gut/Brain Natures.

V Causes of Imbalance

- Overstimulation
- Too many choices
- Overexertion
- Negative emotions
- Irregular routine
- Stressful situations
- Exposure to cold and/or windy weather
- Unpleasant interactions
- Excessive travel

V Results of Imbalance

- Hyperactivity
- Restlessness
- Distraction
- Nervousness
- Heightened emotions
- Forgetfulness
- Anxiousness
- Poor digestion
- Fearfulness
- Constipation
- Loneliness
- Irregular appetite
- Rapid mood changes
- Inability to focus

V Recommendations

- Establish and maintain a daily routine
- Have healthy snacks
- Protect from cold, windy weather
- Avoid video games at night
- Reduce excessive stimulation
- Maintain a fixed bedtime routine
- Make plans and goals
- Minimize the number of choices
- Guard against fatigue
- Engage in creative activities
- Take naps to recharge physically and emotionally

P Causes of Imbalance

- Overheating
- Not eating on time
- Hot spices such as chilies
- Stimulating TV, video games
- Not enough cool liquids

- Overly competitive situations
- Negative emotions

P Results of Imbalance

- Irritability
- Intense hunger
- Impatience
- Excessive thirst
- Anger
- Sensitivity to spicy and/or fried foods
- Being critical
- Indigestion and/or heartburn
- Aggression or hostility
- Excessive perspiration
- Jealousy
- Hot temper
- Obsessive-compulsive behaviors

P Recommendations

- Eat on time, especially lunch
- Exercise regularly but don't overdo it
- Swimming and water sports to cool and balance
- Prevent overheating
- Keep the air conditioner running
- Drink plenty of cooling liquids
- Avoid spicy foods

K Causes of Imbalance

- Excessive sleep
- Overeating
- Too little activity
- Exposure to hot, humid weather
- Lack of mental stimulation
- Exposure to cold, damp weather
- Lack of regular exercise

K Results of Imbalance

- Stubbornness
- Sadness
- Depression
- Withdrawal
- Lethargy
- Excess mucus
- Laziness
- Weight gain

K Recommendations

- Keep mentally and physically stimulated
- Try a dehumidifier
- If it's damp and cold, have warm drinks
- Include exercise in your routine
- Try not to overeat; light meals are best
- Volunteering can build nurturing bonds
- Welcome new relationships—get out and meet people
- Be easy about adapting to change

Remember:

- **Be Prevention Oriented**

- **Stick To A Good Daily Routine**

- **Be Aware Of Subtle Changes In Your Mind And Emotions**

- **Listen To Your Body, Especially During The Change Of Seasons. This Will Help Prevent Imbalances And Illness**

CHAPTER 22

Lifestyle Guidelines

Digestion

1. Food is regarded as medicine.

2. Digestion is critical for every aspect of your health.

3. Eat your main meal at noon when the digestive power of *agni* is highest.

4. Avoid cold water (especially with ice) right before, during, and after a meal. *It reduces the fire of digestion.* Instead, sip small amounts of room-temperature or warm water with your meal. Warm water with a squeeze of lemon is not only tasty, but excellent for your digestion.

5. *Always sit* when you eat.

6. *Avoid stimulation*, such as the TV, telephone, or heated emotional conversations at the table.

7. Enhance your digestion by *remaining seated* for about five minutes after you have finished eating. This sounds strange and may feel peculiar at first, but after a while you'll get to like it. (Your stomach will thank you in many ways.)

8. *Make sure to take enough time to digest one meal before starting the next.*

9. The freshness and purity of food is very important. It is better to eat organic food than ingest toxins like man-made pesticides and fertilizers in every bite.

10. Probiotics can be helpful for many people and have been shown to reduce symptoms of IBS.

11. Discover your own Nature and learn which foods and spices are best for you according to Ayurveda.

12. Periodically use the Rest and Repair Diet to improve your gut health and reboot your microbiome.

Daily Routine

1. Get up early and drink 8 ounces of water. The water shouldn't be cold. You can leave a glass of water by your bedside overnight and drink it first thing in the morning.

2. Reduce stress through the practice of meditation. (We recommend twice-daily practice of the Transcendental Meditation technique.)

3. Exercise according to your Gut/Brain Nature, and practice yoga regularly.

4. Get to bed before 10:00 pm and get enough sleep each night.

Meditation

Studies have shown that the Transcendental Meditation technique produces unique changes that are different from other meditation techniques.

Research shows that it reduces blood pressure and helps people with heart disease. The American Heart Association states: "The Transcendental Meditation technique is the only meditation practice that has been shown to lower blood pressure." Other quotes from this same statement include:

> "Because of many negative studies or mixed results and a paucity of available trials, all other meditation techniques (including MBSR or *mindfulness-based stress reduction*) received a 'Class III, no benefit, Level of Evidence C' recommendation. Thus, other meditation techniques are not recommended in clinical practice to lower BP at this time."

> "Transcendental Meditation practice is recommended for consideration in treatment plans for all individuals with blood pressure > 120/80 mm Hg."

> "Lower blood pressure through Transcendental Meditation practice is also associated with substantially reduced rates of death, heart attack, and stroke."

Research shows that TM practice reduces other cardiovascular risk factors such as cholesterol levels and tobacco use, and it also helps to improve certain at-risk conditions such as metabolic syndrome. In addition, meditators exhibit an improved ability to adapt to stressful situations and a marked decrease in levels of plasma cortisol, commonly known as the "stress hormone." Studies in other areas of health show improvements in such conditions as asthma, insomnia, pain, and alcohol and drug abuse, as well as reduced anxiety and improved mental health.

A five-year study on some two thousand individuals showed that TM practitioners use medical and surgical health care services approximately one-half as often as other insurance users. This study was conducted in cooperation with Blue Cross–Blue Shield and controlled for other factors that might affect health care use, such as cost sharing, age, gender, geographic distribution, and profession.

In Québec, Canada researchers compared the changes in physician costs for TM practitioners with those of non-practitioners over a five-year period. After the first year, the TM group's health care costs decreased 11%, and after five years, their cumulative cost reduction was 28%. The TM patients also required fewer referrals, resulting in lower medical expenses for tests, prescription drugs, hospitalization, surgery, and other treatments.

Recent research has revealed that the TM practice changes the expression of genes in the DNA. Studies show that TM affects the expression of over seventy genes and increases the expression of a particular gene which could help reverse the aging process.

Many studies document how TM can slow and even reverse the aging process. Long-term TM meditators have been shown to have a biological age that is roughly twelve years younger than their non-meditating counterparts. Researchers at Harvard University studied the effects of TM on mental health, behavioral flexibility, blood pressure, and longevity in residents of homes for the elderly. The TM group had significant improvements in cognitive functioning and blood pressure as compared to the control groups. Even more notable, all members of the TM group were still alive three years after the program began, in contrast to about only half of the members of the control group.

In one five-year study conducted at the Medical College of Wisconsin in Milwaukee, as we mentioned before, the TM group had a 48% risk reduction in heart attacks, strokes, and deaths as compared to randomly assigned controls.

Exercise and Yoga

Specific exercise are recommended for each Gut/Brain Nature.

Vatas tend to be quick and excel at short bursts of exercise, but they must always be careful not to strain. A twenty to thirty minute walk every day, and stretching exercises like yoga or dance are very good for us. (People with a combination VP Nature often make excellent professional dancers.)

Pittas are naturally more athletic and can do more strenuous exercises. However, their competitive nature can get them into trouble if they exercise too intensely. Pittas have to be careful not to overdo it. Swimming is beneficial for all types, and especially for Pittas since the water has a cooling effect on their hot Pitta nature.

Kaphas need regular exercise more than any of the other types, especially given their tendency to gain weight. They are well suited to exercise that involves stamina and endurance. Some of the world's finest athletes are a combination of Kapha and Pitta Natures. Their Kapha part balances and grounds them, while the Pitta part gives them speed and accuracy.

Nose Breathing

According to Ayurveda, the best way to breathe during exercise is Nose Breathing. You will discover that it's almost impossible to do Nose Breathing when you are pushing yourself too hard. Discomfort during this kind of breathing is a signal that you are overexerting and need to make an adjustment. Begin by walking slowly; close your mouth and easily inhale and exhale through your nose. Walking on level ground is best at first. Later, you can walk on a gradually increasing slope, which will challenge you a little more—but only when you're ready. If you feel the need to breathe through your mouth at any time, this is a signal for you to slow down, breathe as you ordinarily would, and take a rest. In a couple of weeks, you will find it quite easy to breathe only through your nose and you will be able to take longer, deeper breaths.

When your nose breathing becomes effortless, it will help to keep you balanced and centered while you are engaged in action. If you can't breathe through your nose, by all means, take in a soft breath through your mouth. Nose Breathing takes time to adjust to, especially while you are walking or engaged in activity or sport. Remember, the second your breathing begins to feel difficult or forced, inhale through your nose and out through your mouth for a little while before you try pure Nose Breathing again. It's important for older people (or for anyone out of shape) to build up your nose breathing practice very slowly. Scientific studies show that nose breathing directly affects key centers in the brain, which have to do with emotions and thinking.

Yoga

Yoga has long been recognized as a method to improve and maintain your body while you are on the path to health, happiness, success, fulfillment, and, ultimately, enlightenment. Research has revealed that yoga postures improve certain psychological conditions, including anxiety and depression, and provide health benefits for those with high blood pressure, various pain syndromes, and immune disorders.

Choose whichever form of yoga best suits your individual nature, age, and needs. We recommend the Maharishi Yoga Asana program because it is especially respectful of your body and your consciousness, and supports the experience of transcendence.

Optional One Day Detox Cleanse

This simple cleanse helps to detox your body and re-establish balance in your Gut/Brain Nature, especially if you have a predominance of Pitta. Check with your doctor before doing any cleanse.

- Get up early (6:00 or 7:00) on a weekend morning when you can rest the entire day.

- Mix two tablespoons of castor oil with half a cup of orange juice.

- Drink the mixture (castor oil by itself can sometime make a person gag and the citrus makes it easier to get down).

- For the rest of the day have only liquid meals: bone broth, soup, freshly squeezed juices, or a protein shake.

- Take it easy (no strenuous exercise) and make sure a toilet is nearby.

- In a few hours you will usually begin to have bowel movements (sometimes sudden and explosive), which can vary in number from 2-3 to (in rare cases) 8-10.

- Go to be early and make sure to have a light breakfast the next morning.

- It may take 24 hours to resume regular bowel movements.

Skin Care and Essential Oils

My wife, former Vogue model Samantha Jones, and I wrote a book called *Deep Beauty*—a user-friendly introduction to Ayurveda that focuses on your skin and which essential oils work best for you. The book provides a quiz to determine your True Skin Type, or TST, and explains why knowing your True Skin Type is an extraordinary guide to caring for your skin, your health, and your inner and outer beauty at any age.

After reading *Deep Beauty*, you will be able to look at the label of any skin product and understand the most essential facts about the contents:

- *Does it contain oils that are good for my particular skin?*

- *Are the oils listed worth the price?*

- *Are there chemicals I should check for toxicity?*

Children and Parenting

Dharma Parenting: Understand Your Child's Brilliant Brain for Greater Happiness, Health, Success, and Fulfillment, by Dr. Robert Keith Wallace and Dr. Fredrick Travis, helps you understand how to use both contemporary science and ancient Ayurvedic knowledge to raise a happy and successful child. The word "dharma" means a way of living that upholds the path of evolution, maintains balance, and supports both prosperity and spiritual freedom.

The first tool of *Dharma Parenting* is to determine your child's—and your own—brain/body type through a simple quiz. The brain/body type is similar to the Gut/Brain Nature. It helps you understand why one child learns quickly and forgets quickly while another learns slowly and forgets slowly; why one child is hyperactive and another is calm and steady; or why one falls asleep quickly while another takes hours to fall asleep. *Dharma*

Parenting offers unique insight into areas of universal parental concern such as: emotions, behavior, language, learning styles, diet, health, and, most importantly, the parent-child relationship.

Successful Aging and the Cycles of Life

According to Ayurveda, there are three main stages of life, which are based on the three doshas, Vata, Pitta and Kapha. The Kapha quality predominates in all children during the first part of life, regardless of one's individual nature. This is good for growth and gives a sense of contentment and happiness, and if your childhood situation isn't so good, the Kapha time of life serves as a sort of cushion to help you get through the tough times.

As you grow out of childhood, you enter the middle, or Pitta, stage of life. This is a more capable and responsible time, when you accomplish bigger things and may start a family.

Finally, at about the age of 60, everyone enters the last and most sensitive Vata period of life. Many problems can arise during this period, both as a result of getting older and because Vata imbalances become much more common.

To live longer, Ayurveda recommends:

- Follow the Ayurvedic guidelines for better digestion

- Eat according to your Gut/Brain Nature

- Exercise regularly according to your Gut/Brain Nature

- Follow an Ayurvedic daily routine

- Learn to practice Transcendental Meditation

- Be Happy

Neurophysiology of Transformation

How do you make a change or transformation in your life? Change usually requires a certain degree of energy. You must be prepared to take a new path that might conflict with your current preferences. This means overcoming existing habits and even addictions that can be deeply rooted in your physiology and neurochemistry.

Numerous experiments clearly show that *experience changes the brain*. When you learn to play a new musical instrument, for example, certain areas in the motor cortex become thicker. Your brain is incredibly dynamic, with new synapses and pathways formed constantly. These new pathways are, in turn, supported by molecular changes in neurons and supporting cells, which may be initiated by changes in the expression of specific genes.

Behavioral changes can also be influenced by your gut bacteria. You have learned how your gut bacteria may play an important role in weight gain or loss, and can even influence the brain pathways involved in eating disorders and in alcohol and drug addiction.

So how do you make a change? Take a simple example: say you are overweight and want to lose a few pounds. You might simply want to look better or you may need to lose weight because your doctor tells you that obesity is a primary risk factor for diabetes and heart disease.

Is this motivation enough? Well, it begins the process. The next step is for you to start to make some changes in your life. If you are immersed in bad habits or addictions, change may require the rewiring of specific circuits or networks in your brain and the rebooting of your microbiome. Some habits have been reinforced since early childhood so the neural networks and physiological patterns in your body have been present for a long period of time.

Sometimes one change stimulates others. For example, if you learn to meditate or begin an exercise program, it's then easier to stop smoking or lose weight. Ayurveda suggests that in the beginning, you make small changes very slowly, and understand that it will take time before the change "sticks." If you consider that your habits are based on neural circuits in the brain, or a disruption in your microbiome, then you realize that these are physical systems that take time to change. You have to create new alternative circuits in your brain, and you have to heal your gut lining and reboot your microbiome.

We have offered you some of the basic tools so that you can take steps forward in this process of change. And we encourage and support you in your journey of transformation to a new level of health and happiness. Please take advantage of every health resource available to you, but remember that food is medicine and you will make a huge difference in every aspect of your mental and physical health simply by making changes in your eating habits and lifestyle.

Lifestyle Guidelines

AFTERWORD

Maharishi University of Management (MUM) is accredited by the North Central Association of Colleges and Schools and has outstanding programs to train health coaches in Maharishi AyurVeda and Integrative Medicine.

Your Healthy Gut is an online course, offered through MUM's Continuing Eduation Program, which carefully guides you through *The Rest And Repair Diet*. We invite you to visit the MUM website at mum.edu and explore these remarkable opportunities.

ACKNOWLEDGMENTS

We would like to thank the great people who have contributed to *The Rest And Repair Diet*:

George Foster for his brilliant cover and for formatting and illustrating the book;

Andrew Stenberg for his Ayurvedic contribution to the diet program;

Dr. Jim Davis for his expert medical advice;

Alexis Farley for her delicious recipes;

Ted and Danielle Wallace for their feedback and support;

Nicole Windenberg, Rick Nakata, and Fran Clark for editing and proofreading; Allen Cobb for graphics.

ABOUT THE AUTHORS

ROBERT KEITH WALLACE is a pioneering researcher on the physiology of consciousness. His work has inspired hundreds of studies on the benefits of meditation and other mind-body techniques, and his findings have been published in *Science, American Journal of Physiology,* and *Scientific American.* After receiving his BS in physics and his PhD in physiology from UCLA, he conducted postgraduate research at Harvard University.

Keith currently serves as Professor and Chairman of the Department of Physiology and Health, and is a Trustee at Maharishi University of Management (MUM) in Fairfield, Iowa. Dr. Wallace has written a number of books and given hundreds of lectures around the world.

SAMANTHA JONES WALLACE was once featured on the cover of *Vogue, Cosmopolitan,* and *Look.*

Happily married for over forty years, the Wallaces have a combined family of four children and six grandchildren.

Samantha's passions include painting, exploring essential oil skin care, and creating rare organic perfume. A longtime practitioner of Transcendental Meditation, she also has a deep understanding of Ayurveda and its relationship to health and wellbeing.

Samantha is the coauthor of *Gut Crisis,* and *Quantum Golf,* and is an editor of *Dharma Parenting.* Her most recent book, *Deep Beauty,* is a friendly introduction to Ayurveda with a special emphasis on essential oil skin care.

ANDREW STENBERG is a Senior Graduate Faculty of Maharishi University of Management (MUM), researching and teaching the Maharishi AyurVeda approach to health, longevity, and happiness. He holds a Master's degree in Maharishi Vedic Science.

As a Vedic Health Educator in Australia, Andrew had his own Maharishi AyurVeda (MAV) practice with over 11,000 consultations. He was also Senior Lecturer at Maharishi Vedic College, Melbourne, Australia, from 1996 to 2001, training health professionals in Maharishi AyurVeda.

DR. JIM DAVIS is Associate Professor in the Physiology and Health Department, and the Medical Director of the Integrative Wellness Center at Maharishi University of Management (MUM). He provides clinical experience for undergraduate and graduate students studying Maharishi AyurVeda.

Dr. Davis graduated from the Texas College of Osteopathic Medicine in Ft. Worth Texas and was trained in Maharishi AyurVeda at MUM. He has been in General Practice for 31 years focusing primarily on Osteopathic Manual Medicine and Maharishi AyurVeda.

ALEXIS FARLEY is passionate about food! She learned to cook in her grandma's kitchen, and after graduating from the University of Calgary, visited over 30 countries, experiencing the foods and flavors of different cultures. Returning to Vancouver, BC, Alexis became a chef at a boutique bed and breakfast and began her journey of helping people heal through diet and lifestyle. Most recently, she was a chef at an organic farm and yoga retreat in Northern California. Alexis' expertise is creative plant-based cooking, in which food is medicine and ingredients showcase themselves, leaving guests nourished and energized.

NOTES AND REFERENCES

Chapters 1-4

Gut Crisis: How Diet, Probiotics, and Friendly Bacteria Help You Lose Weight and Heal Your Body and Mind by Robert Keith Wallace, PhD and Samantha Wallace, Dharma Publications, 2017

See our website: https://docgut.com.

Chapter 5

Conlon, MA and Bird, AR, The Impact of Diet and Lifestyle on Gut Microbiota and Human Health. *Nutrients* 2015; 7, 17-44

O'Sullivan, A et al., The Influence of Early Infant-Feeding Practices on the Intestinal Microbiome and Body Composition in Infants. *Nutrition and Metabolic Insights* 2015; 8(S1) 1–9

Clarke, SF et al., Exercise and associated dietary extremes impact on gut microbial diversity. *Gut* Dec 2014; 63(12):1913-20

Wegienka, G et al., The Role of the Early-Life Environment in the Development of Allergic Disease. *Immunololgy and Allergy Clinics of North America* 2015; 35(1):1-17

Chapter 6

References for different Ayurveda constitutions

Travis, FT and Wallace, RK, Dosha brain-types: A neural model of individual differences. *Journal of Ayurveda and Integral Medicine* 2015; 6, 280-85

Dharma Parenting: Understand your Child's Brilliant Brain for Greater Happiness, Health, Success, and Fulfillment by Robert Keith Wallace, PhD, and Fred Travis, PhD, Tarcher/Perigee, 2016

Maharishi Ayurveda and Vedic Technology: Creating Ideal Health for the Individual and World, Adapted and Updated from The Physiology of Consciousness: Part 2 by Robert Keith Wallace, PhD, Dharma Publications, 2016

Dey, S and Pahwa, P, Prakriti and its associations with metabolism, chronic diseases, and genotypes: Possibilities of newborn screening and a lifetime of personalized prevention. *Journal of Ayurveda and Integral Medicine* 2014; 5:15-24

Vernocchi, P et al., Gut Microbiota Profiling: Metabolomics Based Approach to Unravel Compounds Affecting Human Health. *Frontiers in Microbiology* 2016; 7:1144

Arumugam, M et al., Enterotypes of the human gut microbiome. *Nature* 2011, 473,174-180

Chauhan, NS et al., Western Indian Rural Gut Microbial Diversity in Extreme Prakriti Endo-Phenotypes Reveals Signature Microbes. *Frontiers in Microbiology* 2018; 9:118.

References for biorhythms

Reynolds, AC et al., The shift work and health research agenda: Considering changes in gut microbiota as a pathway linking shift work, sleep loss and circadian misalignment, and metabolic disease. *Sleep Medicine Reviews* 2017; 34:3-9

Paulose, JK et al., Human Gut Bacteria Are Sensitive to Melatonin and Express Endogenous Circadian Rhythmicity. *PLoS ONE* 2016; 11(1): e0146643

Voigt, RM et al., Circadian Rhythm and the Gut Microbiome. *Cell* 2016; 161(1): 84-92

Zarrinpar, A et al., Daily Eating Patterns and Their Impact on Health and Disease. *Trends in Endocrinology and Metabolism* 2016; 27(2):69-83

Thaiss, CA et al., Trans-kingdom control of microbiota diurnal oscillations promotes metabolic homeostasis. *Cell* 2014; 159(3): 514-29

Summa, KC and Turek, FW, Chronobiology and Obesity: Interactions between Circadian Rhythms and Energy Regulation. *Advances in Nutrition* 2014; 5: 312S–319S

Deckle-Mahan, K and Sassone-Corsi, P, Metabolism and the Circadian Clock Converge. *Physiological Reviews* 2013; 93(1): 107–135

Konturek, PC et al., Gut clock: implication of circadian rhythms in the gastrointestinal tract. *Journal of Physiology and Pharmacology* 2011; 62(2):139-50

Davenport, ER et al., Seasonal Variation in Human Gut Microbiome Composition. PLoS ONE 2014; 9(3): e90731.

References for prebiotics and bastis

Peterson, CT et al., Therapeutic Uses of *Triphala* in Ayurvedic Medicine. *Journal of Alternative and Complementary Medicine* 2017; 23(8):607-614

Oliva, S et al., Randomised clinical trial: the effectiveness of Lactobacillus reuteri ATCC 55730 rectal enema in children with active distal ulcerative colitis. *Alimentary Pharmacology and Therapeutics* 2012; 35: 327–334

Periasamy, S et al., Sesame oil accelerates healing of 2,4,6-trinitrobenzenesulfonic acid-induced acute colitis by attenuating inflammation and fibrosis. *Journal of Parenteral and Enteral Nutrition* 2013; 37(5):674-82

Hou, RC et al., Increase of viability of entrapped cells of Lactobacillus delbrueckii ssp. bulgaricus in artificial sesame oil emulsions. *Journal of Dairy Science* 2003; 86(2):424-8.

Matthes, H et al., Clinical Trial: probiotic treatment of acute distal ulcerative colitis with rectally administered Escherichia coli Nissle 1917 (EcN). *BMC Complementary and Alternative Medicine* 2010; 10:13

For information on Transcendental Meditation:

An Introduction to Transcendental Meditation: Improve Your Brain Functioning, Create Ideal Health, and Gain Enlightenment Naturally, Easily, Effortlessly by Robert Keith Wallace, PhD, and Lincoln Akin Norton, Dharma Publications, 2016

Transcendental Meditation: A Scientist's Journey to Happiness, Health, and Peace, Adapted and Updated from The Physiology of Consciousness: Part I by Robert Keith Wallace, PhD, Dharma Publications, 2016

The Neurophysiology of Enlightenment: How the Transcendental Meditation and TM-Sidhi Program Transform the Functioning of the Human Body, by Robert Keith Wallace, PhD, Dharma Publications, 2016

See website https://www.TM.org

Chapter 7

The Brain Maker: The Power of Gut Microbes to Heal and Protect Your Brain For Life by David Perlmutter and Kristin Loberg, Little, Brown and Company, 2015

Grain Brain: The Surprising Truth about Wheat, Carbs, and Sugar— Your Brain's Silent Killers by David Perlmutter and Kristin Loberg, Little, Brown and Company, 2013

Eat Dirt: Why Leaky Gut May Be the Root Cause of Your Health Problems and 5 Surprising Steps to Cure It by Dr. Josh Axe, Harper Wave, 2016

Fat for Fuel: A Revolutionary Diet to Combat Cancer, Boost Brain Power, and Increase Your Energy by Dr. Joseph Mercola, Hay House, Inc.; 1 edition, 2017

Chapter 8

Fetissov, SO, Role of the gut microbiota in host appetite control: bacterial growth to animal feeding behaviour, *Nature Reviews Endocrinology* 2017: 13, 11–25

The Prime: Prepare and Repair Your Body for Spontaneous Weight Loss by Dr. Kulreet Chaudhary, Harmony, 2016

Braniste, V et al., The gut microbiota influences blood-brain barrier permeability in mice. *Science Translational Medicine* 2014; 6(263):263ra158

Diana, M, The Dopamine Hypothesis of Drug Addiction and Its PotentialTherapeutic Value. *Frontiers in Psychiatry* 2011; 2:64

Chapter 9

See Wikipedia for more details about the South Pole expedition.

Chapter 10

Li, X and Atkinson, MA, The role of gut permeability in the pathogenesis of type 1 diabetes—a solid or leaky concept? *Pediatric Diabetes* 2015; 7, 485-92

Fat for Fuel: A Revolutionary Diet to Combat Cancer, Boost Brain Power, and Increase Your Energy by Dr. Joseph Mercola, Hay House, Inc.; 1 edition, 2017

Gluten Freedom: The Nation's Leading Expert Offers the Essential Guide to a Healthy, Gluten-Free Lifestyle by Alessio Fasano, MD, Wiley; 1 edition, 2014

Fasano, A, Intestinal permeability and its regulation by zonulin: diagnosis and therapeutic implications. *Clinical Gastroenterology and Hepatology* 2012; 10,1096-100

Fasano, A, Zonulin, Regulation of tight junctions, and autoimmune diseases. *Annals of the New York Academy of Sciences* 2012; 1258(1):25-33

Sturgeon, C and Fasano A, Zonulin, a regulator of epithelial and endothelial barrier functions, and its involvement in chronic inflammatory diseases. *Tissue Barriers* 2016;4(4):e1251384.

Groschwitz, KR and Hogan, SP, Intestinal Barrier Function: Molecular Regulation and Disease Pathogenesis. *The Journal of Allergy and Clinical Immunology* 2009; 124(1):3-22

Bischoff, SC et al., Intestinal permeability – a new target for disease prevention and therapy. *BMC Gastroenterology* 2014; 14:189

Viggiano, D et al., Gut barrier in health and disease: focus on childhood. *European Review for Medical and Pharmacological Sciences* 2015; 19, 6, 1077-1085

Chapter 11

Tillisch, K, et al., Brain structure and response to emotional stimuli as related to gut microbial profiles in healthy women. *Psychosomatic Medicine.* 2017; Oct;79(8):905-913

Tillisch, K, et al., Consumption of Fermented Milk Product With Probiotic Modulates Brain Activity. *Gastroenterology* 2013; 144(7).

Carabotti, M et al., The gut-brain axis: interactions between enteric microbiota, central and enteric nervous systems. *Annals of Gastroenterology* 2015; 28, 203-209

Mu, C et al., Gut Microbiota: The Brain Peacekeeper. *Frontiers in Microbiology.* March 2016; 7, 345

Konturek, PC et al., Stress and the gut: pathophysiology, clinical consequences, diagnostic approach and treatment options. *Journal Of Physiology And Pharmacology* Dec 2011; 62(6):591-9

Million, M and Larauche, M, Stress, sex, and the enteric nervous system. *Journal of Neurogastroenterology and Motility* 2016; 28: 1283–1289

Roohafza, H et al., Anxiety, depression and distress among irritable bowel syndrome and their subtypes: An epidemiological population based study. *Advanced Biomedical Research* 2016; 5:183.

Spiller, R, Serotonin and GI clinical disorders. *Neuropharmacology* 2008; 55:1072–80

Atkinson, W et al., Altered 5-hydroxytryptamine signaling in patients with constipation and diarrhea-predominant irritable bowel syndrome. *Gastroenterology* 2006; 130:34–43

Dunlop, SP et al., Abnormalities of 5-hydroxytryptamine metabolism in irritable bowel syndrome. *Clinical Gastroenterology and Hepatology* 2005; 3:349–57.

Cani, PD and Knauf, C, How gut microbes talk to organs: The role of endocrine and nervous routes. *Molecular Metabolism* 2016; 5(9):743-752.

Chapter 12

Gut and Psychology Syndrome by Dr. Natasha Campbell-McBride, MD, Medinform Publishing Cambridge, UK, 2010

Sarkar, A et al., Psychobiotics and the Manipulation of Bacteria–Gut–Brain Signals. *Trends in Neurosciences* November 2016; 39, (11), 763–781

Evrensel, A and Ceylan, ME. The Gut-Brain Axis: The Missing Link in Depression. *Clinical Psychopharmacology and Neuroscience* 2015; 13(3): 239-244.

Magnusson, KR et al., Relationships between diet-related changes in the gut microbiome and cognitive flexibility. *Neuroscience* Aug 2015; 300:128-40.

Chaidez, V et al., Gastrointestinal problems in children with autism, developmental delays or typical development. *Journal of Autism and Developmental Disorders* 2014; 44(5):1117-1127

Krajmalnik-Brown, R et al., Gut bacteria in children with autism spectrum disorders: challenges and promise of studying how a complex community influences a complex disease. *Microbial Ecology in Health and Disease* 2015; 26:10.3402/mehd.v26.26914

Hsiao, EY et al., Microbiota modulate behavioral and physiological abnormalities associated with neurodevelopmental disorders. *Cell* 2013; 155:1451–63

Buffington, SA et al., Microbial Reconstitution Reverses Maternal Diet-Induced Social and Synaptic Deficits in Offspring. *Cell* Jun 2016; 165(7):1762-75

Parracho, H et al., A Double-Blind, Placebo-Controlled, Crossover-Designed Probiotic Feeding Study In Children Diagnosed With Autistic Spectrum Disorders, *International Journal of Probiotics and Prebiotics* 2010; 5, 2, 69-74

Braniste, VA et al., The gut microbiota influences blood-brain barrier permeability in mice. *Science Translational Medicine* 2014;6(263):263ra15

Chapter 13

Ghoshal, UC et al., Small Intestinal Bacterial Overgrowth and Irritable Bowel Syndrome: A Bridge between Functional Organic Dichotomy. *Gut and Liver* 2017; 11(2):196-208

Pinto-Sanchez, MI et al., Probiotic Bifidobacterium longum NCC3001 Reduces Depression Scores and Alters Brain Activity: a Pilot Study in Patients With Irritable Bowel Syndrome. *Gastroenterology* 10.1053/j. gastro.2017; 05.003

Kennedy, PJ et al., Irritable bowel syndrome: A microbiome-gut-brain axis disorder? *World Journal of Gastroenterology* 2014; 20(39): 14105–14125

Chedid, V et al., Herbal therapy is equivalent to rifaximin for the treatment of small intestinal bacterial overgrowth. *Global Advances in Health and Medicine* 2014; 3(3):16-24.

Brown, K et al., Efficacy of a Quebracho, Conker Tree, and M. balsamea Willd blended extract in patients with irritable bowel syndrome with constipation. *Journal of Gastroenterology and Hepatology Research* 2015; 4:1762–1767.

Brown, K et al., Response of irritable bowel syndrome with constipation patients administered a combined quebracho/conker tree/M. balsamea Willd extract. *World Journal of Gastrointestinal Pharmacology and Therapeutics* 2016; 7(3):463-468

The Complete Low-FODMAP Diet: A Revolutionary Plan for Managing IBS and other Digestive Disorders by Sue Shepherd, PhD and Peter Gibson, MD, first published by Penguin, 2011 and then The Experiment, 2013

Ahmed, I et al., Microbiome, Metabolome and Inflammatory Bowel Disease. *Microorganisms* 2016; 4, 20

Narushima, S et al., Characterization of the 17 strains of regulatory T cell-inducing human-derived Clostridia. *Gut Microbes* May/June 2014; 5:3, 333–339

Konig, J et al., Consensus report: faecal microbiota transfer – clinical applications and procedures. *Alimentary Pharmacology and Therapeutics* 2017; 45: 222–239

Chu, ND et al., Profiling Living Bacteria Informs Preparation of Fecal Microbiota Transplantations. Zoetendal EG, ed. *PLoS ONE* 2017; 12(1):e0170922

Vermeire, SJ et al., Donor species richness determines faecal microbiota transplantation success in inflammatory bowel disease.*Journal of Crohn's and Colitis* 2016; 10: 387–94

Van Nood, E et al., Duodenal infusion of donor feces for recurrent Clostridium difficile. *New Engl and Journal of Medicine* 2013; 368(5): 407–15

Chapter 14

Lin, J et al., Probiotics supplementation in children with asthma: A systematic review and meta-analysis. *Journal of Paediatrics and Child Health.* Sep 2018;54(9):953-961

Cuello-Garcia, CA et al., Probiotics for the prevention of allergy: a systematic review and meta-analysis of randomized controlled trials. *Journal of Allergy and Clinical Immunology* 2015; 136(4):952–61

Ridaura, VK et al., Gut microbiota from twins discordant for obesity modulate metabolism in mice. *Science* Sep 2013; 341(6150):1241214

Pluznick, JL et al., Olfactory receptor responding to gut microbiota-derived signals plays a role in renin secretion and blood pressure regulation. *Proceedings of the National Academy of Sciences* 2013; 110 (11) 4410-4415

de Brito Alves, JL et al., New Insights on the Use of Dietary Polyphenols or Probiotics for the Management of Arterial Hypertension. *Frontiers in Physiology* 2016; 7:448

Robles-Vera, I et al., Antihypertensive Effects of Probiotics. *Current Hypertension Reports* Apr 2017; 19(4):26

Fu, J et al., The Gut Microbiome Contributes to a Substantial Proportion of the Variation in Blood Lipids. *Circulation Research* 2015; 117:817-824

Musso, G et al., Obesity, Diabetes, and Gut Microbiota: The hygiene hypothesis expanded? *Diabetes Care* 2010; 33(10):2277-2284

Tuovinen, E et al., Cytokine response of human mononuclear cells induced by intestinal Clostridium species. *Anaerobe* 2013; 19(1)

Marijon, E et al., Rheumatic heart disease. *Lancet* 2012; 379 (9819): 953–64

Festi, D et al., Gut microbiota and metabolic syndrome. *World Journal of Gastroenterology* November 2014; 21; 20(43): 16079-16094

Sevelsted, A et al., Cesarean Section and Chronic Immune Disorders. *Pediatrics* January 2015; 135,1

Brand, HV et al., Increased risk of allergic rhinitis among children delivered by cesarean section: a cross-sectional study nested in a birth cohort. *BMC Pediatrics* 2016; 16:57

Houghteling, PD and Walker, WA, From birth to "immuno-health", allergies and enterocolitis. *Journal of Clinical Gastroenterology* 2015; 49(0 1):S7-S12

Campbell, AW, Autoimmunity and the Gut. *Autoimmune Diseases* 2014; 2014:152428

Benakis, C et al., Commensal microbiota affects ischemic stroke outcome by regulating intestinal γδ T cells. *Nature Medicine*, 2016; 22(5):516-23

Pascal, M et al., Microbiome and Allergic Diseases. *Frontiers in Immunology* 2018; 9:1584.

For information on clinical trials go to: https://clinicaltrials.gov/ and enter "fecal microbiome transplant" and "probiotics" in the search box.

Chapter 15

Does Sugar Cause Inflammation in the Body? by Mary Jan Brown, Healthline, November, 2016

Inflammatory Claims about Inflammation by Jeff Schweitzer, Huffington Post, May, 2015

Silbernagel, G et al., Plasminogen activator inhibitor-1, monocyte chemoattractant protein-1, e-selectin and C-reactive protein levels in response to 4-week very-high-fructose or -glucose diets. *European Journal of Clinical Nutrition* 2014 Jan; 68(1):97-100

Kuzmua, JN et al., No differential effect of beverages sweetened with fructose, high-fructose corn syrup, or glucose on systemic or adipose tissue inflammation in normal-weight to obese adults: a randomized controlled trial. *American Journal of Clinical Nutrition* 2016; 104:306–14

The Case Against Sugar by Gary Taubes, Knopf, 2016

Lustig, RH, Sugar the Bitter Truth, YouTube video

Lustig, RH, Sickeningly Sweet: Does Sugar Cause Type 2 Diabetes? Yes. *Canadian Journal of Diabetes* 2016 Aug;40(4):282-6.

Miriam, B et al., Added Sugars and Cardiovascular Disease Risk in Children: A Scientific Statement From the American Heart Association, *Circulation.* 2017 May 09; 135(19): e1017–e1034

Serena, G et al., The Role of Gluten in Celiac Disease and Type 1 Diabetes. *Nutrients* 2015 Aug 26;7(9):7143-62

Leonardi, GC et al., Ageing: from inflammation to cancer. *Immunity and Ageing* 2018; 15:1

Chapter 16

The Danger of Dairy: https://www.mindbodygreen.com

Bordoni, A et al., Dairy products and inflammation: A review of the clinical evidence, *Critical Reviews in Food Science and Nutrition* 2017; 57:12, 2497-2525

Lordan, R et al., Dairy Fats and Cardiovascular Disease: Do We Really Need to be Concerned? *Foods* 2018, 7(3), 29

Drouin-Chartier, JP et al., Comprehensive Review of the Impact of Dairy Foods and Dairy Fat on Cardiometabolic Risk. *Advances in Nutrition* 2016; 7(6):1041-1051

Lordan, R and Zabetakis, I, Invited review: The anti-inflammatory properties of dairy lipids. *Journal of Dairy Science* 2017; 100(6):4197-4212

Telle-Hansen, VH et al., Does dietary fat affect inflammatory markers in overweight and obese individuals?—a review of randomized controlled trials from 2010 to 2016. *Genes and Nutrition* 2017;12:26

General figures of lactose intolerance are given in Wikipedia: https://en.wikipedia.org/wiki/Lactose_intolerance

Reference for milk allergy

Bahna SL, Cow's milk allergy versus cow milk intolerance. *Annals of Allergy, Asthma and Immunology* 2002; 89:6(1): 56–60

Reference for casein and beta casomorphin

Casein: https://en.wikipedia.org/wiki/Casein and Kost, NV et al., Beta-casomorphins-7 in infants on different type of feeding and different levels of psychomotor development. *Peptides* 2009 Oct; 30(10):1854-60

References for the A1 verses A2 controversy

Truswell, AS, The A2 milk case: a critical review, European Journal of Clinical Nutrition, 2005; 59 (5): 623–631European Food Safety Authority, Review of the potential health impact of β-casomorphins and related peptides. *EFSA Journal* 2009; 7 (2): 231r

Pal, S et al., Milk Intolerance, Beta-Casein and Lactose. *Nutrients* 2015; 7(9): 7285-7297

Jianqin, S et al., Effects of milk containing only A2 beta casein versus milk containing both A1 and A2 beta casein proteins on gastrointestinal physiology, symptoms of discomfort, and cognitive behavior of people with self-reported intolerance to traditional cows' milk. *Nutrition Journal* 2016; 15:35

Jianqin, S et al., Erratum to: 'Effects of milk containing only A2 beta casein versus milk containing both A1 and A2 beta casein proteins on gastrointestinal physiology, symptoms of discomfort, and cognitive behavior of people with self-reported intolerance to traditional cows' milk'. *Nutrition Journal* 2016; 15:45

He, M et al., Effects of cow's milk beta-casein variants on symptoms of milk intolerance in Chinese adults: a multicentre, randomised controlled study. *Nutrition Journal* 2017; 16:72

Brooke-Taylor, S et al., Systematic Review of the Gastrointestinal Effects of A1 Compared with A2 β-Casein, *Advances in Nutrition*, 2017; 8: 5, (1) 739–748

Chapter 17

http://news.gallup.com/poll/184307/one-five-americans-include-gluten-free-foods-diet.aspx

Leonard, MM et al., Celiac Disease and Nonceliac Gluten Sensitivity: A Review. *Journal of the American Medical Association* 2017 Aug 15; 318(7):647-656

Fasano, A et al. Nonceliac gluten and wheat sensitivity. *Gastroenterology* 2015; 148(6):1195-204.

Catassi, C et al., Diagnosis of Non-Celiac Gluten Sensitivity (NCGS): The Salerno Experts' Criteria. *Nutrients* 2015; 7(6):4966-4977.

Catassi, C et al., The Overlapping Area of Non-Celiac Gluten Sensitivity (NCGS) and Wheat-Sensitive Irritable Bowel Syndrome (IBS): An Update. *Nutrients* 2017; 9(11): 1268.

Dalla Pellegrina, C et al., Effects of wheat germ agglutinin on human gastrointestinal epithelium: insights experimental model of immune/epithelial cell interaction. *Toxicology and Applied Pharmacology* 2009 Jun 1; 237(2):146-53.

Rubio-Tapia, A et al., Increased prevalence and mortality in undiagnosed celiac disease. *Gastroenterology* 2009 Jul; 137(1):88-93.

Ludvigsson, JF et al., Small-intestinal histopathology and mortality risk in celiac disease. *Journal of the American Medical Association* 2009 Sep 16; 302(11):1171-8.

Fasano, A, Physiological, pathological, and therapeutic implications of zonulin-mediated intestinal barrier modulation: living life on the edge of the wall. *American Journal of Pathology* 2008 Nov; 173(5):1243-52.

Hollon, J et al., Effect of gliadin on permeability of intestinal biopsy explants from celiac disease patients and patients with non-celiac gluten sensitivity. *Nutrients* 2015 Feb 27; 7(3):1565-76.

Zevallos, VF et al., Nutritional Wheat Amylase-Trypsin Inhibitors Promote Intestinal Inflammation via Activation of Myeloid Cells. *Gastroenterology* 2017 Apr;152(5):1100-1113.e12.

Schuppan, D and Zevallos V., Wheat amylase trypsin inhibitors as nutritional activators of innate immunity. *Digestive Diseases Journal* 2015; 33(2):260-3.

Schuppan, D et al., Non-celiac wheat sensitivity: Differential diagnosis, triggers and implications. *Best Practice and Research Clinical Gastroenterology* 2015; 29(3):469-76.

Junker, Y et al., Wheat amylase trypsin inhibitors drive intestinal inflammation via activation of toll-like receptor 4. *Journal Of Experimental Medicine* 2012; 209(13):2395-408.

Saja, K et al., Activation dependent expression of MMPs in peripheral blood mononuclear cells involves protein kinase A. *Molecular and Cellular Biochemistry* 2007 Feb; 296(1-2):185-92.

Cinova, J et al., Role of Intestinal Bacteria in Gliadin-Induced Changes in Intestinal Mucosa: Study in Germ-Free Rats. Leulier F, ed. PLoS ONE. 2011; 6(1)

Laparra, JM and Sanz Y, Bifidobacteria inhibit the inflammatory response induced by gliadins in intestinal epithelial cells via modifications of toxic peptide generation during digestion. *Journal of Cellular Biochemistry* 2010; 109: 801–7

Fernandez-Feo, M et al., The Cultivable Human Oral Gluten-Degrading Microbiome and its Potential Implications in Celiac Disease and Gluten Sensitivity. *Clinical Microbiology and Infection* 2013 Sep; 19(9): E386–E394.

Grain Brain: The Surprising Truth about Wheat, Carbs, and Sugar—Your Brain's Silent Killers by David Perlmutter and Kristin Loberg, Little, Brown and Company, 2013

Eat Wheat: A Scientific and Clinically-Proven Approach to Safely Bringing Wheat and Dairy Back Into Your Diet by Dr. John Douillard, Morgan James Publishing, 2017

Chapter 18

Pinto-Sanchez, MI et al., Probiotic Bifidobacterium longum NCC3001 Reduces Depression Scores and Alters Brain Activity: a Pilot Study in Patients With Irritable Bowel Syndrome. *Gastroenterology.* 2017. doi: 10.1053/j.gastro.2017.05.003.

Kennedy, PJ et al., Irritable bowel syndrome: A microbiome-gut-brain axis disorder? *World Journal of Gastroenterology* Oct 2014; 20(39): 14105–14125

Wilkins, T et al., Probiotics for Gastrointestinal Conditions: A Summary of Evidence. *American Family Physician* Aug 2017; 96:3,170-178

Zmora, N et al., Personalized Gut Mucosal Colonization Resistance to Empiric Probiotics Is Associated with Unique Host and Microbiome Features. *Cell* 2018; 174, 6,1388-1404

Suez, J et al., Post-Antibiotic Gut Mucosal Microbiome Reconstitution Is Impaired by Probiotics and Improved by Autologous FMT *Cell* 2018; 174, 6,1406-1423

Chapter 19

Bredesen, DE et al. Reversal of cognitive decline in Alzheimer's disease. *Aging* 2016; 8(6):1250-1258. doi:10.18632/aging.100981.

Bredesen, DE, Metabolic profiling distinguishes three subtypes of Alzheimer's disease. *Aging* 2015; 7(8):595-600.

The End of Alzheimer's: The First Program to Prevent and Reverse Cognitive Decline by Dale Bredesen, MD, Avery, 2017 and website (https://www.drbredesen.com/)

Chapter 20

See online programs for Master of Science in Maharishi Ayurveda and Integrative Medicine at mum.edu

Chapter 21

See quiz at https://docgut.com

Chapter 22

References on Transcendental Meditation:

Wallace R.K. Physiological effects of Transcendental Meditation. *Science* 1970; 167:1751-1754

Wallace, RK et al., A wakeful hypometabolic physiologic state. *American Journal of Physiology* 1971; 221(3): 795-799

Dillbeck, MC and Orme-Johnson DW, Physiological differences between Transcendental Meditation and rest. *American Psychologist* 1987; 42:879–881

Travis, FT and Shear, J, Focused attention, open monitoring and automatic self-transcending: Categories to organize meditations from Vedic, Buddhist and Chinese traditions. *Consciousness and Cognition* 2010; 19(4):1110-1118

Schneider, RH, et al., Stress Reduction in the Secondary Prevention of Cardiovascular Disease: Randomized, Controlled Trial of Transcendental Meditation and Health Education in Blacks. *Circulation: Cardiovascular Quality and Outcomes* 2012; 5:750-758

Jayadevappa, et al., Effectiveness of Transcendental Meditation on functional capacity and quality of life of African Americans with congestive heart failure: a randomized control study. *Ethnicity and Disease* 2007; 17: 72-77

Castillo-Richmond, A, et al. Effects of the Transcendental Meditation Program on carotid atherosclerosis in hypertensive African Americans, *Stroke* 2000; 31: 568-573

Kondwani, K et al., Left Ventricular Mass Regression with the Transcendental Meditation Technique and a Health Education Program in Hypertensive African Americans. *Journal of Social Behavior and Personality* 2005; 17:181-200

Brook, RD et al., Beyond Medications and Diet: Alternative Approaches to Lowering Blood Pressure. A Scientific Statement from the American Heart Association. *Hypertension* 2013; 61(6):1360-83

Anderson, JW, et al., Blood pressure response to Transcendental Meditation: a meta-analysis. *American Journal of Hypertension* 2008; 21 (3): 310-316

Barnes, VA, et al., Impact of Transcendental Meditation on ambulatory blood pressure in African-American adolescents. *American Journal of Hypertension* 2004; 17: 366-369

Rainforth, MV, et al., Stress reduction programs in patients with elevated blood pressure: a systematic review and meta-analysis. *Current Hypertension Reports* 2007; 9:520–528

Cooper, MJ et al., Transcendental Meditation in the management of hypercholesterolemia. *Journal of Human Stress* 1979; 5(4): 24–27

Royer, A, The role of the Transcendental Meditation technique in promoting smoking cessation: A longitudinal study. *Alcoholism Treatment Quarterly* 1994; 11: 219-236

Paul-Labrador, M et al., Effects of randomized controlled trial of Transcendental Meditation on components of the metabolic syndrome in subjects with coronary heart disease. *Archives of Internal Medicine* 2006; *166*:1218-1224

Wilson, A et al., Transcendental Meditation and asthma. *Respiration* 1975; 32:74-80

Gaylord, C et al., The effects of the Transcendental Meditation technique and progressive muscle relaxation on EEG coherence, stress reactivity, and mental health in black adults. *International Journal of Neuroscience* 1989; 46: 77-86

Haratani, T et al., Effects of Transcendental Meditation (TM) on the mental health of industrial workers. *Japanese Journal of Industrial Health* 1990; 32: 656

Alexander, C.N., et al. Treating and preventing alcohol, nicotine, and drug abuse through Transcendental Meditation: A review and statistical meta-analysis. *Alcoholism Treatment Quarterly* 11: 13-87, 1994.

Eppley, KR et al., Differential effects of relaxation techniques on trait anxiety: A meta-analysis. *Journal of Clinical Psychology* 1989; 45: 957-974

Orme-Johnson, DW and Barnes, VA, Effects of the Transcendental Meditation technique on Trait Anxiety: A Meta-Analysis of Randomized Controlled Trials. *Journal of Alternative and Complementary Medicine* 2013; 19: 1-12

Orme-Johnson, DW, Medical Care Utilization and the Transcendental Meditation Program. *Psychosomatic Medicine* 1987; 49: 493–507

Orme-Johnson, DW and Herron RE, An Innovative Approach to Reducing Medical Care Utilization and Expenditures. *American Journal of Managed Care* 1997; 3: 135–144

Herron, RE et al., The Impact of the Transcendental Meditation Program on Government Payments to Physicians in Quebec. *American Journal of Health Promotion* 1996; 10: 208–216

Herron, RE, and Hillis, SL, The Impact of the Transcendental Meditation Program on Government Payments to Physicians in Quebec: An Update. *American Journal of Health Promotion* 200014(5): 284–291

Herron, RE, Can the Transcendental Meditation Program Reduce the Medical Expenditures of Older People? A Longitudinal Cost-Reduction Study in Canada. *Journal of Social Behavior and Personality* 2005; 17(1): 415–442

Herron, RE, Changes in Physician Costs Among High-Cost Transcendental Meditation Practitioners Compared with High-Cost Non-practitioners Over 5 Years. *American Journal of Health Promotion* 2011; 26(1): 56–60

Duraimani, S. et al., Effects of Lifestyle Modification on Telomerase Gene Expression in Hypertensive Patients: A Pilot Trial of Stress Reduction and Health Education Programs in African Americans. *PLOS ONE* 2015; 10(11): e0142689,

Wenuganen, S, Anti-Aging Effects of the Transcendental Meditation Program: Analysis of Ojas Level and Global Gene Expression. Maharishi University of Management, *ProQuest Dissertations Publishing*, 3630467, 2014

Glaser, JL et al., Elevated serum dehydroepiandrosterone sulfate levels in practitioners of the Transcendental Meditation (TM) and TM-Sidhi programs. *Journal of Behavioral Medicine* 1992; 15: 327-341

Wallace, RK et al., The effects of the Transcendental Meditation and TM-Sidhi program on the aging process. *International Journal of Neuroscience* 1982; 16: 53-58

Barnes VA et al., Impact of Transcendental Meditation on mortality in older African Americans—eight year follow-up. *Journal of Social Behavior and Personality* 2005; 17(1): 201-216

Schneider, RH et al., Long-term effects of stress reduction on mortality in persons > 55 years of age with systemic hypertension. *American Journal of Cardiology* 2005; 95: 1060-1064

Alexander, CN et al., Transcendental Meditation, mindfulness, and longevity. *Journal of Personality and Social Psychology* 1989; 57: 950-964

Alexander, CN et al., The effects of Transcendental Meditation compared to other methods of relaxation in reducing risk factors, morbidity, and mortality. *Homeostasis* 1994; 35: 243-264

References on exercise and yoga:

Zelano, C et al., Nasal Respiration Entrains Human Limbic Oscillations and Modulates Cognitive Function. Journal of Neuroscience December 2016; 36 (49) 12448-12467

https://www.mum.edu/yoga

Cramer, H et al., Is one yoga style better than another? *Complementary Therapies in Medicine* 2016 Apr;25:178-87

Woodyard, C, Exploring the therapeutic effects of yoga and its ability to increase quality of life. *International Journal of Yoga* 2011 Jul-Dec; 4(2): 49–54.

Streeter, CC et al., Effects of yoga versus walking on mood, anxiety, and brain GABA levels: a randomized controlled MRS study. *Journal of Alternative and Complementary Medicine* 2010 Nov; 16(11):1145-52. doi: 10.1089/acm.2010.0007. Epub 2010 Aug 19.

Ross, A and Thomas, S, The Health Benefits of Yoga and Exercise: A Review of Comparison Studies. *The Journal of Alternative and Complementary Medicine* 2010; 16: 1, 3–12.

Reference on Parenting:

Dharma Parenting: Understand Your Child's Brilliant Brain for Greater Happiness, Health, Success, and Fulfillment by Robert Keith Wallace, PhD and Fredrick Travis, PhD, Tarcher Perigee, Penguin Random House, 2016

Reference on skin care and essential oils:

Deep Beauty by Samantha Wallace and Robert Keith Wallace, PhD, Dharma Publications, in press

Additional websites

https://docgut.com

https://doshaguru.com

https://dharmaparenting.com

https://deepbeautybook.com

APPENDIX 1

Products Used in Diet

See **https://docgut.com** for Maharishi Ayurveda Products:

Digest and Detox Tea
Digest Tone Triphala Plus
Ashwagandha
Brahmi
Vata, Pitta, and Kapha Organic Tea
Vata, Pitta, and Kapha Organic Churna Spice Mix

See **www.banyanbotanicals.com** for Kitchari Spice Mix.

APPENDIX 2

The Maharishi Integrative Ayurveda Institute offers educational programs and expert health coaches who can help you create an integrative health plan with Maharishi AyurVeda®. See **www. maharishi-ayurveda.us** for more details, particularly on qualified health coaches for *The Rest And Repair Diet*.

Index

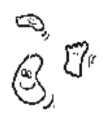

CPSIA information can be obtained
at www.ICGtesting.com
Printed in the USA
BVHW030208200720
584109BV00001B/44